The White Coat Investor's
Guide for Students

WHY YOU SHOULD READ THIS BOOK

Way back in 1999 I enrolled as a student at The University of Utah School of Medicine. The years in medical school were four of the best years of my life. I thoroughly enjoyed nearly every minute of it. Life was good. I married my college girlfriend the month before classes began and our children were still half a decade away. We were living at the base of the Wasatch Mountains where I spent afternoons rock climbing, mountain biking, or skiing. I was finally studying something that would have a direct effect on what I was going to be doing for the rest of my life.

Compared to years of slogging through difficult subjects while competing with neurotic pre-meds for top grades, medical school felt downright casual. (Maybe a little too casual given my grade on the first gross anatomy test.) We were on an honors-pass-fail grading system and the only "gunning" going on was to be one of the first MS1s who could beat a team of MS2s on the foosball table. After attending a large high school and an even larger university, my class of 100 students actually provided an opportunity to get to know most of my classmates on an individual level.

From the first few weeks of medical school, I developed an intense admiration for my colleagues. Later in my career, I discovered that I loved to teach and help medical students in any way I could. One of the first things we did when The White Coat Investor became financially successful was to start the White Coat Investor Scholarship Program. It was our way of giving back. One reason I admire these students is their dedication and idealism. I had the opportunity to serve on the admissions committee as an MS4. Given the caliber of people applying to our school, I was shocked that there had been room for me!

I cringe every time I see a medical or dental student become a little more cynical. I hate seeing doctors advise pre-meds and even their own children to avoid medicine or dentistry. These are wonderful professions that still command respect, provide opportunities to help people on the worst days of their lives, and, eventually, provide a good standard of living. However, there is a serious, worsening problem in our medical and dental schools and it needs to be addressed.

The problem is that medical and dental students are making some of the most significant financial decisions of their lives without the basic financial literacy they need to make the decisions properly. For the most part, the schools themselves are not providing it. In fact, in some respects, the schools have a conflict of interest in providing it since they are at least part of the problem, but more on that later.

Consider the major decisions with financial consequences that are often made before you will complete your training:

- Whether and whom you marry
- Whether you stay married
- Whether you have children
- What profession you choose
- Where you go to school
- How you pay for that school
- How much money you borrow
- How you manage those loans
- Which specialty you choose
- Where you train for that specialty
- Whether you go into academics or private practice
- What area of the country you practice in
- Whether you are an employee or an owner of your job
- Whether or not you insure yourself and your family against the loss of your ability to practice medicine or even your own death
- How expensive of a house you live in
- What you drive
- How much you spend on your lifestyle including vacation and entertainment expectations

The most important year in a physician's financial life is that first year out of training when the "big bucks" (i.e. an attending physician's paychecks) start rolling in. Due to the critical importance of that year, a great deal of my writing and work at The White Coat Investor has been targeted at graduating residents and new attendings. Unfortunately, as the cost of education rises, many doctors are already in a massive hole by the time they reach that point. Time and time again I have heard doctors tell me "I wish I would have learned this in school!" or ask "Where were you 10 years ago?" or "Why doesn't anybody teach this in dental school?"

My first book, *The White Coat Investor: A Doctor's Guide to Personal Finance and Investing* was designed as a general guide for doctors at any stage of training. My second book, *The White Coat Investor's Financial Boot Camp: A 12-Step High-Yield Guide to Bring Your Finances Up to Speed* was aimed squarely at that target demographic of graduating residents and new attendings. This book, however, is aimed at you—a medical or dental student. While the book will contain a small amount of information about managing finances as a resident and some general financial literacy information, the vast majority of it is designed to help you avoid the mistakes that your predecessors have made during school.

By reading and applying the lessons here, you will:

- Know whether or not your education was a good investment,
- Graduate from school with as little debt as possible,
- Know exactly how to manage those student loans,
- Quit feeling guilty about borrowing money to pay for school, and
- Be prepared to achieve the financial success you expected when you were accepted to school.

If you are like I was in medical school, you do not think too much about finances and are willing to practice your craft practically for free. You did not sign up to do this for the money and actually find it alarming to discover that many doctors 10 years ahead of you feel underpaid and stressed about money. I am convinced that a financially secure doctor is a better partner, spouse, parent, and clinician. Financially secure doctors spend more time at home and bring home less stress. They can provide the best care for their patients without having to worry about making payroll or their next student loan or mortgage payment. They have more patience with colleagues and coworkers. They can practice in a way that provides the best care without having to spend precious time and energy worrying about money.

If you are already a financial whiz, this book will provide you a few doctor-specific tips that help you optimize your efforts. If you are like most students and know little to nothing about personal finance and investing, spending a few hours with this book will likely be worth millions of dollars to you over the course of your life.

That money by itself is not necessarily valuable. After all, most of the time it will just look like numbers on a computer screen. However, if you use it properly, those account balances can purchase your freedom—freedom to create the life you most desire without regard to financial concerns.

You CAN do this. You are a smart person and a hard worker. It is time to stop worrying about your financial situation.

You CAN understand the basics of earning, saving, investing, spending, and giving money.

You CAN pay off your debts rapidly after school and build a secure financial future that allows you to focus on your family and patients and even buy a few luxuries along the way.

Let's get started!

PRAISE FOR GUIDE FOR STUDENTS

I wish I had this information when I was a student. This book should be required reading as part of the dental and medical school curriculum.
    –Alexandra E. Forest, DDS, MD

An invaluable resource for pre-med students, medical students, and those in residency.
    –Rick Ferri, CFA

Succinct summary of financial gems!
    –Col. Gregory Morgan, Ret. USAF, CPA

This book provides solid financial advice for anyone in medical school or anyone considering medical school. More importantly, it provides a foundational framework for making sound and prudent financial decisions throughout one's life. It is worth its weight in gold.
    –Ryan Kelly, CFP

Dr. Dahle has changed my approach to handling money, loans, and financial planning. His book is packed full of straightforward practical recommendations and is a must-read for medical students!
    –Mitchell D. Belkin, Medical Student

This should be the required textbook for a Financial Literacy 101 course in every medical and dental school curriculum. This book will teach you how to become financially independent by making smart moves with your money as a student, a resident, and as a practicing doctor or dentist.
    –Angela Chiara, Dental Student

This book should be read once a year during medical education training to keep your financial future on a path to success.
    –Warner Weber

The one book to read the summer before starting medical school.

–Jake Babel, Medical Student

How I wish I had this amazing book when I started school. I would be in a very different place now financially.

–Jonathan Polak, MD

Great advice from an author that is easy to understand and relatable. I do not know why talking about this stuff has almost become taboo in the profession. Imagine "First Aid for the USMLE" but for your financial freedom. A very important read for health professions in the midst of medical training.

–Austin C. Snyder, Medical Student

Dr. Dahle did it again. The breadth of financial topics covered in concise, easy-to-read chapters makes this book an excellent "go-to" for medical students and residents who want to understand the basics of personal finance quickly and learn how to practically apply economic concepts to every step of their medical journey.

–Chelsea G. Swanson, JD

Dr. Dahle has changed my approach to handling money, loans, and financial planning. His book is packed full of straightforward, practical recommendations and is a must-read for medical students!

–Mitchell D. Belkin, Medical Student

This is the book that I wish I had read before I had applied to dental school. It is a high-yield guide for prospective medical and dental students so that they can make good financial decisions and focus on taking care of their patients rather than having to fret about their finances.

–Chris Roff, Dental Student

Dahle does a great job of providing concise, practical information for the pre-health undergraduate, medical student, or resident who has recognized the importance of financial stewardship. If you are wondering how a med school choice, student loans, and eventual career choice might affect your future, this book is essential preventative medicine for your financial wellbeing.

–J. Lee Rawlings, MD

Dr. Dahle has outdone himself. This book is a blueprint for financial success for medical school and beyond. A must-read for every medical and dental student!

–Mujtaba A. Hameed, Medical Student

Dr. Dahle's succinct, accessible, and high-yield financial pearls are a must-have for every medical and dental student in the nation. His lessons power readers to build the life they want to build.

–Nicholas P. Cozzi, MD, MBA

This book contains everything I wish I had learned in my last year of dental school. It is an invaluable resource for any MD/DMD to help in the monumental decisions awaiting them during and immediately after their professional training.

–Dr. Craig and Ashley Weinstein

Also by James M. Dahle, MD

The White Coat Investor:
A Doctor's Guide to Personal Finance and Investing

The White Coat Investor's Financial Boot Camp:
A 12-Step High-Yield Guide to Bring Your Finances Up to Speed

The White Coat Investor's

Guide for Students

How Medical and Dental Students Can Secure Their Future

James M. Dahle, MD

ISBN: 978-0-9914331-2-4

Limitation of Liability: This publication is designed to provide accurate and authoritative information in regard to the subject matter covered. It is sold with the understanding that neither the author nor the publisher is engaged in rendering legal, accounting, or other professional service. If legal advice or other expert assistance is required, the services of a competent professional should be sought. Neither the author nor the publisher shall be liable for any loss of profit or any other commercial damages, including but not limited to special, incidental, consequential, or other damages.

Cover Design: Ashley Chandler
Book Design: Emily Macbean
Author Photograph Credit: Taylor Cutchen

Published in the United States of America

To the doctors
who have cared for and will care for my family and friends

FOREWORD

There is a saying on Wall Street that if you really want to get to know someone, you either marry them or manage their money. I have only been married once and do not plan on changing wives after 40 years. When people ask me if gold is a good investment, I point to my wedding ring and tell them it was the best investment I ever made. I hope you are as lucky.

I have had a humble and gratifying 30-year career getting to know thousands of investors and working with them on their personal finances. Many of my clients were and are physicians and dentists. Some became self-made decamillionaires by 45 years old, and some will be working well into their 70s before they have enough to retire. Most are somewhere in the middle.

If you are reading this, you are probably not a doctor or dentist yet, but someday you will be, and you will earn a good income. But high income alone does not guarantee financial success or even personal solvency. You may be shocked to learn that doctors have one of the highest personal bankruptcy rates, and each year more have trouble keeping their finances straight due to changes brought on by government regulation, decreasing insurance reimbursements, and rising malpractice costs.

What causes one doctor to become rich and another to stay poor? There is no correlation between the medical or dental school you attend and whether you will accumulate $20 million or only $500,000 by the time you retire. The type of medicine you practice does not matter either; every specialty pays enough to retire comfortably if you manage your money properly. Location does not matter either; I have worked with doctors and dentists who live in remote parts of the country who have a large nest egg, and those who live in high-income areas and barely have a dime to their name.

You will be well trained during school and residency, but the important money and finance lessons you will need to reach financial independence are not taught in these programs. Nor will you learn them by attending free chicken dinners put on by financial advisors and insurance salespeople who will hound you for the rest of your life. Do not think for a moment that watching Jim Cramer scream into a camera like a deranged parent yelling at a ref while watching their 10-year-old play soccer will give you any answers either.

What does make a difference? The key is self-learning. Going out and finding sources of information that lead you to good money habits. This is what every financially successful doctor has done. Unfortunately, this is not an easy task. You must be very selective about what you read and who you listen to because the world is full of con artists and you are a primary mark. This is a big problem for the medical community, and one that Dr. Jim Dahle has been addressing for two decades.

I met Jim many years ago at a Bogleheads annual conference. The Bogleheads (*www.bogleheads.org*) are a not-for-profit, person-to-person, online community of like-minded individuals who follow the wisdom of John C. Bogle, founder of the Vanguard group of mutual funds.

Jim was a bright, young, ambitious Air Force physician who had been burned by a financial advisor. This led him on a self-education quest with the primary goal of not being taken advantage of again. He made learning about personal finance his passion and was eager to share what he learned with other young doctors. In 2011, he launched *The White Coat Investor* blog and shortly after published his first book by the same name. Since then Jim has added more books, a podcast, videos, online courses, and an annual Physician Wellness and Financial Literacy Conference.

This book is unique because it addresses the financial needs of medical school students and those in residency, as well as money issues you will face when you go into the world and begin practice. It is a "soup to nuts" guide of practical advice that is worth its weight in gold.

As an investment advisor who has seen things go right for doctors and dentists, and has seen things go horribly wrong, my contribution to the book is this: If you do what Dr. Dahle recommends during school, training, and your first 10 years in practice, then you can live like most doctors cannot for the rest of your life.

Finally, I honor your commitment to medicine. It is not an easy profession. The hours are long and the responsibility is great. But the world needs smart people like you to take care of the rest of us, and you are to be commended for your decision. You also deserve just rewards for your efforts, whatever you choose them to be.

Good luck!

Rick Ferri, CFA

President, The John C. Bogle Financial Literacy Center

CONTENTS

PART 2 – MANAGING FINANCES DURING RESIDENCY

PART 3 – THE NEXT STEP: ACHIEVING FINANCIAL LITERACY

INTRODUCTION

There is an old joke that involves a parent giving career advice to a child: "I do not care what you choose to do for a living, as long as you become a doctor or a lawyer." For many decades medicine, dentistry, and law have been respected professions in the general community, accomplishing important work and commanding high incomes. In more recent years, the cost of entry to these professions has skyrocketed. While the price of undergraduate college has gone up significantly, the cost of professional school has dramatically outpaced it. Consider the statistics: from the 1985–1986 school year until the 2017–2018 school year, general inflation (i.e. the rise in the cost of goods and services) as measured by the Consumer Price Index (CPI) has been 2.6% per year.[1] The price of college (tuition, fees, room, and board) over that time period has increased at a rate of 5% per year,[2] 2.4% more than the overall rate of inflation. The Association of American Medical Colleges does not track the cost of room and board, but the price of tuition and required fees over that same time period has increased by 7–8.7% per year (less for public in-state students, more for private schools and public out-of-state students),[3] a rate 4.4–6.1% higher than the rate of inflation!

Compound interest is a powerful thing. Over the course of 32 years, compound interest has worked its magic on these seemingly minor annual tuition increases. Even after adjusting for inflation, medical students are now paying four to six times as much for their education! The actual trajectory for dental and law schools is similar, if not worse. Meanwhile, in many ways, the professions have become more difficult. With the dramatic increase in law school seats and the lower bar exam passage rates, it is much harder for attorneys to find any position at all, much less a high paying one. With the consolidation and increasing incorporation of medicine and dentistry, fewer and fewer doctors own their own practices, resulting in lost income potential and control over their work environment. Unsurprisingly, this has led to epidemic proportions of burnout in these professions.

In addition, the percentage of high-income professionals with serious financial problems is increasing rapidly. This was particularly well demonstrated by a recent email I received from a practicing dentist making $102,000 per year who owes $850,000 in student loans. While the physician or dentist with the average income and the average student loan burden is still doing fine, those with above-average student loan burdens and below-average incomes are not. In fact, they might not ever really build wealth at all over the course of their career. According to the annual Medscape Physician Debt and Net Worth Reports,[4] 25% of doctors in their 60s are not millionaires, despite 20–30+ years of physician paychecks. 11–12% of doctors in their 60s have not even acquired a net worth of $500,000!

My goal is that you, dear reader, will not end up as one of these statistics. In fact, I have dedicated a significant portion of my life to helping doctors avoid this tragic fate. I believe that financially secure doctors are better partners (in both senses of the word), parents, and clinicians. Financial insecurity affects patient care. It also affects the make-up of the physician workforce. The rising costs of education prevent those from lower socioeconomic status (heavily skewed toward minorities underrepresented in medicine) from becoming doctors in the first place. During my career, I have not seen much effort to control the rising price of tuition (although there are now a few medical schools that have waived tuition for their students), so I have decided to focus my time and effort at The White Coat Investor on the doctors themselves. If I can help them to become more financially literate and disciplined, perhaps they can be successful with their finances and their practices despite the challenging obstacles placed in their path.

The earlier a doctor obtains the knowledge, skills, and discipline required for success, the more beneficial it will be. Thus you can see the purpose of this book—a book specifically written for the student. Despite the fact that you are still many years away from making "doctor money," now is the time to become smart with money. You simply cannot afford to wait until the "big paychecks" start rolling in to get started learning about money. You will be too far behind at that point, and catching up will require sacrifices that few are willing to make.

I started blogging at *The White Coat Investor* in May of 2011, after years of interacting with doctors on various financial forums on the internet. The blog quickly grew into the most widely-read, physician-specific, personal finance and investing website in the world. I have written literally thousands of blog posts, articles, and emails for people just like you. I have previously written two best-selling books. They are not particularly entertaining, but they have changed the lives of countless doctors. *The White Coat Investor Podcast*, started in 2017, averages 30,000–40,000 downloads per episode. Thousands have taken our online courses. Hundreds of doctors meet together in person every year or two at our live Physician Wellness and Financial Literacy Conference. Tens of thousands follow along on social media and participate in the various online forums we have created and maintain. We have created scholarship programs for students and financial educator awards for their instructors. Our efforts have inspired dozens of other doctors to blog, podcast, write books, and present this information directly to their peers. Through these combined efforts, it is likely that we have indirectly inspired the creation of more wealth by doctors than anyone else on the planet. I say this not to brag, because it has truly been a pleasure to serve such wonderful people, but merely to point out that the simple act of reading this book provides entry into a community of successful professionals who have improved their own lives and the lives of those they care about.

Most of the concepts I teach are not particularly complicated. They are certainly easier to learn than medicine or dentistry. But at the time I started, nobody was teaching these concepts to students, residents, or practicing doctors and the consequences were obvious. If you will learn these principles of financial literacy, apply them in your life, and combine them with your high earning potential, you will rapidly acquire financial security. This will allow you to quit worrying about money. It will also allow you to pay off your debts, build a retirement nest egg, send your children to college, live in a comfortable home, help thousands of patients, travel the world, and eventually reach the point where you do not need to work for money at all. You will find financial freedom, and with that freedom will come a confidence that comes from the knowledge that you do not work for money, money works for you. Money is no longer your master, and you can then afford to take the personal and professional risks in life that will maximize your happiness.

In the first, and most important, section of the book, I am going to teach those financial principles that you can apply right now in medical or dental school to optimize your finances. We will cover the role of money in your career, how to avoid burnout, and how to choose a school. I will discuss the various methods of paying for school and show you how to minimize the cost. I will also eliminate the burden of guilt that many of you feel as a result of living on borrowed money for years. You will learn to live better on less money and to take advantage of government programs and the tax code. You will learn how to choose a specialty and a residency program. Most importantly, you will learn to avoid the financial catastrophes that can start even before you leave school.

The second part of the book is a preparation for the next phase of many of your lives—residency. While the bulk of your time in residency should be focused on learning your craft, there are a few essential financial moves that need to be made to protect you from financial harm and ensure future financial success. We will go over each of these, one by one, in an efficient and high-yield way. I will let you know exactly what you need to do, with none of the fluff. Your time (and mine) is just too valuable for that. We will cover home-buying, student loan management, investing, disability insurance, and life insurance. Mistakes are common in each of these categories, and often cost young doctors tens or even hundreds of thousands of dollars that they do not have. The fewer of these mistakes you make, the better off you will be as you move into your career.

In the final section of the book, I will teach you basic financial literacy with a focus on the financial lives of doctors. You will get to learn about all kinds of interesting, practical subjects that you were probably not taught by your parents, high school, or college. You certainly will not see these subjects in medical school and residency. These include investments, taxes, retirement accounts, financial history, and financial calculations. As if all that is not enough, if you will sign up at *www.whitecoatinvestor.com/bonus*, I will send you four bonus chapters for this book in PDF form that includes important information about financial advisors, insurance, contracts, and real estate investing. You will find this content invaluable as you move into your career. Each bonus chapter is packed with life-changing information you need to know, but nobody at your school is going to teach you.

The information The White Coat Investor offers for someone just like you is priceless as you move forward in your education and career. I encourage you to change your future now. When you sign up for the free bonus chapters, you will also be signed up for our free monthly newsletter, blog posts, and our WCI Boot Camp email series. Sign up with confidence that I will not spam you and you can unsubscribe at any time.

INTRODUCTION

SIGN UP NOW

Acquiring and applying this knowledge early in my career changed my life, and it can change yours. If you do, you will enjoy a career most doctors only dream of. By mid-career, you can eliminate the parts of your job that you dislike. You can drop night shifts and call. You can work with great partners and an ideal patient population. You can go on vacation every month, drive what you wish to drive, and live where you want to live. You can reach financial independence, meaning you will no longer have to work for money and can live solely off your investments. You will not have to check the bank account before buying something you want. You will be able to help family and donate money to charitable causes you support. You may even find that your biggest financial worry is how to instill a work ethic in your children!

You are already doing the hard part. You are taking the steps in your life to ensure that your income will be high enough to provide financial success. However, just achieving that income is no longer enough. You also must minimize the deleterious effects of debt in your life, protect yourself from financial catastrophes, and use your eventual high income to build wealth. I promise you that if you will read and apply the principles you will be introduced to in this book, you will be financially successful. The life you envision is now available to you, but you cannot wait. I frequently receive emails from mid and late-career doctors who wish they had paid more attention to personal finance, investing, and business. The sooner you learn these principles, the sooner they can give you the life you thought you would automatically get when you were accepted into professional school. It might not be automatic, but you can do it. Turn the page and start today.

THE FINANCIALLY SAVVY STUDENT

This section contains the lion's share of this book. If you are a medical or dental student, this book is targeted directly at you. Part one is about your current financial life and contains information that you can put to use right away. We will discuss every aspect of the financial life of a student from the role of money in your career choices to setting you up for later financial success.

There is an old saying that says, "If you can be talked out of medicine, you should be." The truth is most of us who are in medicine could not have been talked out of it no matter the cost or what anyone else said about it. If your experience was like mine, there were many who warned you against going into medicine, citing all of the problems it faces. The problems doctors complained about were different in the 1990s when I was a pre-med student than now, but there have always been problems and it always seems that the "Golden Age of Medicine" ended about five years before you started! These days pre-meds probably worry about going into medicine because of the debt and the burnout.

These are serious issues, but both are manageable, as we will discuss in this section. Medicine is still an incredibly rewarding career. As my friend the private equity manager has frequently told me, "I like my job but at the end of the day I am just making a bunch of rich people richer." As a doctor, you will aid many people as they deal with some of the greatest challenges of their lives, and often interact with them on one of the worst days of their life. You will have a special glimpse into some of the most intimate details of human existence. It is important work, thank you for choosing it.

Now that you have embarked on this path, I want to help you be as successful in it as I can, both professionally and financially

In this section we will discuss how you should think about money, both before and after you graduate from school. We will also talk about how to choose a school and perhaps more importantly, how to pay for it. The importance of thrift, especially while living on loans will be discussed. I include some specific information for the non-traditional student, and will help both physicians and dentists choose a specialty and a residency program. One of the most important parts of this section will be avoiding financial catastrophes. There are a few things you can do early in your career that can really set you back; you should be aware of what they are. Unlike most financial books, we will specifically discuss burnout prevention and treatment. Finally, since most dentists still do not actually attend residency, we will spend a few words advocating for practice ownership as a means of eventually maximizing income.

CHAPTER ONE

WHY MONEY SHOULD NOT BE YOUR PRIMARY MOTIVATION

Medicine and dentistry are fantastic, invigorating callings. You are invited into the most sacred moments of the lives of people you may have just met. Births. Deaths. Illnesses. Injuries. Healings. Betrayals. Frustrations. Relief. Vulnerabilities. You sacrifice one of the best decades of your life to pursue this profession, and consider it an honor. You look forward to the daunting responsibility of caring for others. Yes, it requires sacrifice, but it is worth it.

I used to worry that my work at The White Coat Investor would cause problems in the medical profession. If I taught all doctors how to manage their high income well, maybe they would all retire before age 50 and that would exacerbate the physician shortage and result in worse health for my fellow Americans. I worried that maybe there would be no doctors left to take care of me when I become old and sick! However, after a few years I quit worrying about that for a few reasons:

First, if someone is going to get out of medicine or dentistry just as soon as they have enough money to do so, do we really want that person taking care of us anyway?

Second, lots of doctors, including me, still practice medicine after becoming financially independent. We find it far more enjoyable than when we had to do it. It becomes a well-paid hobby and a labor of love rather than just a source of putting food on the table and a roof over our heads.

Medicine once more becomes the calling we felt drawn to when we applied and interviewed to get into school.

Third, many doctors who take control of their finances have no desire whatsoever to retire early. But their financial know-how allows them to make the career decisions that reduce their burnout and ensure their longevity in the profession. They take sabbaticals, work part-time, go on the "parent track" for a few months or even years, stay in academics, or pursue passion projects.

Fourth, let us be honest. Doctors are people too and just like people everywhere, they find financial information boring. As the old saying goes, "You can lead a horse to water, but you cannot make it drink." No matter how hard I work to get this information into your hands, there will still be plenty of doctors who end up working into their 70s because they cannot afford to retire.

Obviously, I think finances are important and that managing them well can dramatically improve the quality of your life and your ability to help others both at work and outside of work. However, I thought it was important to start this book with a short chapter explaining that despite its importance, it should not be your primary motivation. If you find that it is, perhaps medicine or dentistry is not for you. Let me explain.

You are a smart person. You also know how to work hard. There are other people with those same qualities outside of your profession. A recent study compared Finance, Management, Tech, Law, and Medicine as careers.[5] This study only compared the numbers for "top performers" in each field, but the bottom line was that medicine had the second-lowest salary and the highest debt of the five professions at age 31. If dentistry had been included, it likely would have had the lowest salary and highest debt of the six professions. The truth is that if you want to make a lot of money, there are several better options than medicine or dentistry, despite what your family and friends believe. If someone like you were to put in the time and effort that you will put in as a student and resident into these other fields, you are likely to come out ahead financially.

Even an entrepreneurial pursuit may come out ahead. If you had skipped college and professional school and started working in real estate right out of high school, by the time you reach 30–35 (the age most traditional docs are at the completion of residency) you will likely already be a millionaire and possibly even financially independent. Even a slow-growing side hustle may work out better. Including college, medical school, residency, and years as an attending, 17 years passed before I ever earned more than $200,000 in a year. In 17 years, a serial entrepreneur may have started, built up, and sold three or four separate businesses!

Thus, your motivation to become a doctor needs to be primarily non-financial. When you wrote that personal essay for your application that said you just "love science and want to help people" you better have meant it, or you have already made your first colossal financial mistake (although later in the book, I will talk about how to recover from even this one).

Do not worry. Medicine still provides a great living. I frequently tell medical students that if they cannot live on $200,000–$300,000 per year, they have a spending problem, not an earning problem. They laugh because that truth seems so obvious. Interestingly, doctors 10 years out of residency do not think that line is funny at all, but it is still true. Let us step back from the main point of this chapter for just a moment and consider how easy it is to have a spending problem.

I recall a presentation in medical school demonstrating an ophthalmologist who was earning $300,000 per year and spending $350,000 per year. That is surprisingly easy to do. Consider the hypothetical attending budget below. Not a single line in this budget would be considered outrageous for an attending physician. However, when you put it all together, it adds up to almost twice the average physician income.

Taxes: $140,000

Student Loan Payments: $50,000

College Savings: $25,000

Retirement Savings: $80,000

Mortgage: $40,000

Car Payments: $12,000

Private School Tuition (2 Kids): $36,000

Insurance: $8,000

Utilities: $12,000

Clothing: $4,000

Vacation/Travel: $15,000

Groceries: $12,000

Restaurants: $12,000

Gasoline: $5,000

Auto Repairs/Maintenance: $3,000

Children's Activities: $3,000

Health Insurance: $15,000

HSA Contributions: $7,000

Charity: $20,000

Help for Extended Family: $15,000

Miscellaneous: $10,000

Total: $524,000

I can assure you there are plenty of physicians who make much less than $524,000. Let there be no doubt in your mind that you can spend everything you make as a doctor and then some. Imagine the financial stress that comes from spending $50,000 or even $100,000 more than you make in a given year. It does not have to be like that.

In 2020, the median American household has an income of around $62,000. Most doctors can make twice that working part-time. Another great financial aspect about medicine is that it is still relatively guaranteed. If you gain entrance to medical school, work hard, and do what you are told, you are highly likely to come out the far end of the pipeline with the ability to earn $150,000–$500,000 per year. In business and even other professions, there is far more risk of never obtaining a high income. Unlike medicine or dentistry, just being the average person in the profession does not come with a high income. This trend is probably most concerning in law. While "Big Law" attorneys start out at close to $200,000 per year (while working resident-like hours), the median law school graduate is doing well to have an income similar to that of the median American household.

The fact that you got into medical or dental school does not mean you can ignore money and still expect financial success. The process of becoming a "rich doctor" is relatively simple, but it is not automatic. There are a few things you need to do. By the way, if you do not like the term "rich," feel free to substitute wealthy, comfortable, or financially secure if it makes you feel better. However, building wealth still cannot be your primary motivation. It is not enough to get you through the hours of studying required. It is not enough to get you through the months of clinical training, late nights, loss of sleep, and sacrifices. You will be miserable and you will be a lousy doctor. So make sure your motivations are (at least mostly) pure and spend the time required to become a true expert in your field. Just be sure to carve out a little chunk of time to learn about and take care of your finances too.

MAIN IDEAS

- There are easier ways to make a lot of money than medicine and dentistry.
- You can still earn a comfortable living as a doctor.

ADDITIONAL RESOURCES

- **Blog Post:** Law School for the Rest of Us
  www.whitecoatinvestor.com/law-school-for-the-rest-of-us/

- **Article:** Pay in Banking vs. Consulting vs. Tech vs. Medicine vs. Law
  news.efinancialcareers.com/us-en/3003001/pay-in-banking-vs-consulting-vs-tech-vs-medicine-vs-law

CHAPTER TWO

YOU DO NOT GET A PASS ON MATH

Thank you for dedicating your life to helping other people maintain and recover their health. Just spending time with the seriously injured and ill can be psychologically difficult and can take its toll on you. It is truly noble work, but it does not give you a pass on math.

Medical and dental school is expensive, no matter how you pay for it. The vast majority of medical and dental students did not do any sort of mathematical calculation of the return on investment of using those dollars and that time to acquire a job with a high salary. Becoming a doctor was simply a dream. They could not be talked out of it.

However, just because you have chosen to do something good and noble with your life, you do not get to ignore the financial consequences of your decisions. Dave Ramsey is a radio talk show host who focuses heavily on helping people get out of debt. I do not necessarily always agree with everything he says, and his advice is not always geared toward doctors, but I think it is worth hearing what he said a few years ago after taking a call from a dentist's wife wondering if they should buy a house despite having $480,000 in student loans.

> "Parents this is for you. When you have a 17-year-old and they are very, very bright and they want to be a dentist or a doctor or get a Master's degree or PhD in XYZ, you cannot completely ignore economics because there is a high-income potential

for a certain professional field. Most dentists make $100,000–$150,000. Some dentists have built a practice and they have a business mind in addition to being great dentists and they have a practice that makes them a lot more than that. But they are really the exception. The typical dentist makes $100,000–$150,000. There is absolutely no planet under the sun where the math will work for you to justify going into debt $480,000 to get that job. Stop your children from doing that, if you love them. It is amazing to me that the dumbest thing we do is education—the way we view education, the way we think about education, the way we rationalize and justify ridiculously stupid purchases in education, how dumb we are about education.

It just boggles the mind, the paradox of that. I mean, you would think you would be smart about education, wise about education. Not only do people get these ridiculously dumb degrees and pay $100,000 for them—to get a degree in left-handed puppetry or a PhD in German Polka History or something—and then wonder why they can't make a living. Then they think that the culture owes them forgiveness on their student loans because [they think] you get a pass on math because you're going to be a doctor. You get a pass on math because you're going to be a nurse. You get a pass on math because you're going to be a preacher. You get a pass on math because you're doing this "thing." You don't get a pass on math. Use some sense people. Use some sense. And help your children have some sense. Because some of them don't have any sense."[6]

I agree with Dave that it is foolish to borrow $480,000 to get a job that pays $100,000. The astute reader, however, is currently thinking, "Well how much can I spend to get a job that pays $100,000 or $300,000 and have it actually be a good investment?" As you might imagine, it depends. But let me put out some guidelines, some rules of thumb, that you may find useful.

Most medical and dental students are paying for their education using borrowed money, at least in part. Even if you are paying cash for your education, it is still a good idea to consider the return on investment of your education dollars. However, it is far more critical when you are borrowing money to pay for it.

In 2019, the Association of American Medical Colleges (AAMC) reported that the average senior allopathic (i.e. MD) medical student had a student loan burden of just $200,000.[7] In 2019, the American Association of Colleges of Osteopathic Medicine (AACOM) said that the average osteopathic (i.e. DO) senior medical student reported a student loan total of $265,297.[8] In 2018, the American Dental Education Association (ADEA) stated that the average senior dental student reported a total of $285,184.[9] At these levels of debt and the average physician ($275,000) or dentist ($180,000) income, medical or dental school is still a good investment, even if you borrowed money to pay for it at typical rates. But at higher than average loan burdens and lower than average incomes, that may not be the case.

I prefer to think of this concept as a "debt-to-income ratio" (DTI), a term frequently used in lending. For our purposes today, it is simply the ratio of your total student loans upon completing your training to your expected income upon completing your training.

For example, if you borrow $180,000 to pay for school and that debt grows during residency to $200,000, and then you start a job as a family practitioner that pays $200,000, you would have a DTI of 1, or 1X.

$$\$200,000/\$200,000 = 1$$

At 1X, medical or dental school is an excellent investment. With careful financial management (which we will discuss later in the book), you can pay off that debt within two years of completing your training and then enjoy that high income the rest of your career. I encourage professional students borrowing money to aim for this ratio.

What about a pediatrician making $180,000 who owes $360,000? This person has a 2X ratio. At 2X, the investment was not nearly as good. However, it is probably still an acceptable ratio. With careful financial management, this debt can be cleared within five years of the completion of training.

How about a psychiatrist who borrows $600,000 and then gets a job making $200,000? This person has a 3X ratio. At 3X, things start breaking down. I can no longer describe this decision as a good investment. It does not have a solid return on investment. Unless this doctor figures out a way to boost income significantly, the doc is going to struggle just to get the debt paid off within a decade after finishing training.

Some doctors are at ratios of 4X or worse. I have met a few with seven-figure student loans. A few years back, an orthodontist making $225,000 who owed $1.1 million was featured in the *Wall Street Journal*.[10] At these sorts of ratios, you may never be able to pay off your student loans. The interest alone on a 7% $1,000,000 loan is $70,000 per year. That could easily be ¼, ⅓, or even ½ of your take-home pay. Not paying that interest is even worse. Look how quickly debt compounds at 7%.

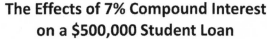

The Effects of 7% Compound Interest on a $500,000 Student Loan

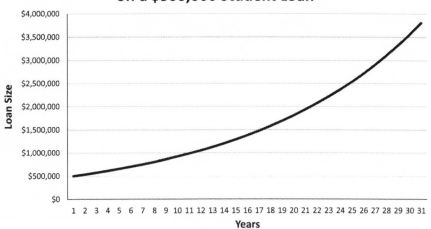

I assure you that you will not feel like a rich doctor with a debt load like that. At those debt loads, you have just a few options and, as you will see later in the book, most of them are not very good. Some of you may be reading this and feeling overwhelmed. Do not abandon ship and close this book. There is hope. Stay with me and we will get to it in a few chapters.

For now, just realize that you do not get a pass on math. As you make decisions on where to attend school, how to pay for it, how well you live as a student, how you manage your student loans, and what field you go into, you need to keep this ratio in mind. If you are going to come out of medical or dental school owing $100,000, the world is your oyster. You can do pretty much anything you want. If you are going to come out owing more than half a million, you need to be very careful both choosing a specialty and choosing your first job after you finish training.

As I told you in the last chapter, money is not everything. It is not even the most important thing. But if you completely ignore it when making career decisions, you are likely to have serious regrets.

MAIN IDEAS

- Medicine and dentistry are still good investments if you can keep your debt to future income ratio below 2.

- You cannot ignore math and finance in making important career decisions.

ADDITIONAL RESOURCES

- **Blog Post:** Maximum Student Loan to Debt Ratio
  www.whitecoatinvestor.com/maximum-student-loan-debt-to-salary-ratio/

- **Blog Post:** Average Medical School Debt
  www.whitecoatinvestor.com/average-medical-school-debt/

- **Survey:** AAMC Graduation Questionnaire
  www.aamc.org/data-reports/students-residents/report/graduation-questionnaire-gq

- **Survey:** AACOM Graduating Class Surveys
  www.aacom.org/reports-programs-initiatives/aacom-reports/entering-and-graduating-class-surveys

- **Survey:** ADEA Senior Student Survey
  www.adea.org/data/seniors/

CHAPTER THREE

HOW TO CHOOSE
A MEDICAL OR DENTAL SCHOOL

This chapter is for the pre-med or pre-dent student. If you are already in school, you can just skip it. It might even make you feel bad to read it. So do not do it. Just go right on ahead to the next chapter.

All right, now that we have run those folks out of here, let me give you the secret to choosing a medical or dental school. It really is not that complicated. Here it is:

Go to the cheapest school you can get into.

Seriously. That is it. That sentence only has nine words but it is full of wisdom. We should discuss all nine of those words. Let us start at the end of the sentence, with the last three words:

Go to the cheapest school you **can get into**.

Many medical and dental students only got into one school. Sometimes that is because they were not strategic about how they applied to schools. Perhaps they did not apply to enough of them. Or maybe they only applied to really competitive schools because they did not get good advice on how competitive they were as an applicant. But more likely, they only got into one school because it is really hard to get into medical or dental school. If you only get into one school, well, go to that school. You might be tempted to take a year off and apply again in hopes of getting into a less expensive school. Do not do that. You might not get in at all. "A bird in the hand is better than two in the bush." You should make your first application your best application and then you know if you only get into one school that you are not likely to do any better next year. But aside from that, the opportunity cost of waiting a year is massive. Maybe you end up in a specialty that makes $400,000 per year. Perhaps $300,000 after tax. So every year you delay starting school you are losing $300,000. The difference in four-year educational costs between the most expensive school in the country and the least expensive school in the country is far less than $300,000 per year.

On a side note, if you do not get into any school at all, it is not necessarily time to give up on your dream. First, make sure it is really your dream. There are plenty of worthwhile, high-paying, fulfilling careers out there that do not involve being accepted to medical, dental, or law school. Second, get some advice from impartial sources, including those in your chosen profession, admissions committee members, and pre-professional advisors. A surprising number of students just did a lousy job of applying. Third, if this really is your career goal and you actually did a fine job of applying, you need to ask yourself if there is something you can do over the next year that will make you a better applicant. If your weakness is a low MCAT score, perhaps intensive study for it will make a difference. If you had a low GPA, perhaps a master's degree or similar coursework can put that concern to rest for admissions committees. If you did not have much exposure to medicine, research, service opportunities, or leadership experience, boost that area of your application. Rewrite your essay, practice interviewing, and consider broadening your application process to include less competitive schools. Be sure to have some fun during this "gap year" too. A year is a long time and there is a lot more to life than your career anyway. It is bad enough to have to be a neurotic pre-med for four years, so I empathize with those who have to do it for five or even six.

Now, let us turn to the first five words in "the secret":

Go to the cheapest school you can get into.

With many things in life, you get what you pay for. However, when it comes to a medical or dental education, most of the time there is very little correlation between the cost of the education and the value of the education. In fact, if there is any correlation at all, it is negative; meaning the more you pay the lower the quality of the education. Quality, of course, is in the eye of the beholder, but in order to introduce some objectivity to the process, let us just consider the main outcome of medical school—matching into residency.

There are three main categories of medical schools that a pre-medical student can attend:

> US MD Schools
>
> US DO Schools
>
> Caribbean MD Schools

In order to compare apples to apples, we will compare the match rate of each of these categories of schools in the MD match. Then we will take a look at the cost of attendance of the schools.

The data on match rates comes from the allopathic (MD) National Residency and Match Program from the 2019 Residency Match.[11] According to the report, the match rates were as follows:

> US MD Schools: 94%
>
> US DO Schools: 85%
>
> Caribbean MD Schools: 59%

Say what you want about discrimination and quality of education, but this is still really the only objective outcome we have to compare these categories to each other. So based on that data, what would you expect to pay to obtain each of these degrees? You would think that it would be most expensive to go to a US MD school and least expensive to go to a Caribbean school, right? But you would be completely wrong.

According to the AAMC, for the 2019–2020 year, the median cost of tuition and fees (including health insurance) at US MD schools was as follows:[12]

> In-State Public: $39,149
>
> Out-of-State Public: $64,807
>
> Private: $62,948

These costs ranged from $0 on the low end to $99,622 on the high end. Obviously, there is a massive difference between paying $39,000 and $100,000 in tuition and fees. All else being equal, a doctor at the most expensive school is likely to leave residency owing at least $200,000 more than the doctor who attended the median in-state public school.

Let us take a look at DO schools:

There are a few public DO schools with in-state tuition similar to that of MD schools, but the vast majority of DO schools are private institutions. According to AACOM, for the 2019–2020 year, the median tuition and fees (NOT including health insurance) are as follows:[13]

> In-State Public: $33,867
>
> Out-of-State Public: $55,361
>
> Private $56,067

Add $5,000–$6,000 for health insurance and you can see that the MD data and the DO data are very similar EXCEPT for the fact that most MD schools are public and most DO schools are private. Because of this effect, the median tuition and fees (again, not including health insurance) at a DO school is $52,800 in-state and $56,067 out-of-state.

As you can see, on average it is going to cost you more to go to a DO school than an MD school, despite the fact that DO seniors have a significantly lower overall match rate. In the most competitive specialties, the DO match rates are much lower.

Finally, we will take a look at Caribbean schools.

These schools confer an MD, but as an "International Medical Graduate" (IMG), a US citizen will have a much harder time matching into a chosen specialty. Almost half of US citizens applying in the US MD match will not match, and that does not account for the fact that many have already chosen not to apply to the more competitive specialties. You would think that a school that only provided a 50/50 chance of helping you get a job would be very inexpensive, right? Not so fast.

There are dozens of these schools on the various islands. The tuition costs and the match rates vary significantly and I know of no central resource that averages them all out. So I will merely provide a convenience sample of some of the schools considered to be "top-notch" Caribbean medical schools. Note that none of these schools actually totals up its annual tuition and fees on its website, for obvious reasons, but if you dig long enough you can find the data.

> St. George's University: $76,354
>
> Ross University: $80,298
>
> American University of the Caribbean: $64,465
>
> Saba University: $49,974

So if we average those four out, we get $67,773. Many students consider these schools "second chance medical schools." You pay more and you have a lower chance of matching.

Note that none of this is to say that you cannot become an exceptional doctor attending a DO or an international medical school. I have known many of both types of doctors in many different specialties that I would trust with my own care and that of my family. But on average, you are going to pay more and have a more difficult time matching.

As you can see, if you are admitted into the average US MD school, US DO school, and Caribbean MD school, choosing the cheaper one is not only going to save you money, but it is usually going to provide a better chance of matching, all else being equal. The education provided to in-state students and out-of-state students at any given school is exactly the same. So if you can get into your state school, that is often your best bet. Some students wonder about the value of one MD school over another, or one DO school over another. There are subtle differences between schools, but they will make a real difference only for a few medical students. Perhaps in a few specialties and for a few academic jobs your choice of medical school will weigh-in significantly. However, for the vast majority of US MD school graduates, the choice of school will have little impact on your match and subsequent career.

For this reason, time and time again you will hear "physicians in the know" advising pre-meds to go to the cheapest school they can get into. Keep in mind when totaling up the cost of a school that you need to include living expenses. It will be much more expensive to attend school in New York City or San Francisco than in Indianapolis or Kansas City.

Occasionally, a medical student gets a scholarship or other type of non-loan financial aid. Obviously, subtract that from the cost of attendance when weighing one school against another.

Dental schools have similar issues. When dentists are asked why they attended a private dental school, the reasons given are frequently financial.

"My state did not have a public dental school."

"I did not get into my state dental school, and the private school is no more expensive than out of state tuition in another state."

"It was the only school I was accepted into."

While there is no official ranking system for dental schools, the Student Doctor Network attempted to rank dental schools using factors such as average DAT score, average GPA, and feedback from those who interviewed there.[14] Of the four schools they gave the top ranking (a "5") to, three were public and one was private. The next category (a "4") included seventeen schools, eleven of which were public. With results like that, it is difficult to argue that private schools are universally better than state schools. The same rule of thumb—attend the cheapest US school you can get into—seems to apply to dentists just as much as physicians.

These principles apply to undergraduate colleges as well. Many medical or dental students bring over $100,000 of debt with them into professional school. It is dramatically easier to cash flow undergraduate school than medical or dental school, especially with proper school selection. You really need to ask yourself how much that "big name" matters, much less the pretty buildings or trees on campus.

Finally, let us look at the most important of the nine words in "the secret":

Go to the cheapest school **you** can get into.

Everybody has a different circumstance. Perhaps there is a very good reason for you to attend a school that is not the very cheapest one on your acceptance list. Perhaps your partner has a job in the city of a slightly more expensive school. Or perhaps the more expensive school has a really unique aspect to their education that you are totally jazzed about or the school name is so prestigious that residency directors and future employers will be impressed, increasing your chances of the career pathway you desire. (Admittedly, this factor will likely become more important for physicians as residency program selection committees adjust to USMLE Step 1 scores only being reported as pass/fail.) Perhaps you just want to live in a big city for a few years. Maybe you are very interested in osteopathic manipulative medicine. There are reasons to violate this rule of thumb, but recognize when you do so that there will be a financial price to pay down the line.

If you are talented enough to be accepted at multiple dental or medical schools, do yourself a favor and attend the one that will cost you the least.

MAIN IDEAS

- The price you pay for your schooling will have significant effects on your future financial life.

- Give serious consideration to attending the least expensive school that accepts you.

ADDITIONAL RESOURCES

- **Blog Post:** Public vs. Private Education Is the Wrong Question
  www.whitecoatinvestor.com/public-versus-private-education/

- **Blog Post:** Is Medical School Still Affordable?
  www.whitecoatinvestor.com/is-medical-school-still-affordable/

CHAPTER FOUR

HOW TO PAY FOR PROFESSIONAL SCHOOL

Your medical or dental education is likely the most expensive purchase of your life thus far. Many graduating professional students have student loan burdens larger than the average American's net worth at retirement. As we saw in our earlier chapter on how to choose a medical or dental school, you need to make a wise decision. Once the decision is made it is time to get down to the nuts and bolts of actually paying for school. There are many options:

PAY CASH

The first option will seem crazy to many readers of this book, but obvious to some of you. If you (or more likely your family) have the money to pay for school, just pay for it. Investing in yourself and your future income is one of the best uses of your money. Given the relatively high professional student loan interest rates, avoiding those loans provides a guaranteed "return" much higher than anything else you can get from a similarly risky investment like a treasury bond or certificate of deposit. Not only do you save the interest, but you save any fees associated with the loans and all of the time, hassle, worry, and student loan advisory fees.

Even if you cannot pay for the entire education, if you have money in a savings account, taxable investing account, or dedicated education account such as a 529 or Coverdell Education Savings Account (ESA), plan to use it. There are two guiding principles as far as how to use the money. The first principle is to avoid the least attractive student loans whenever possible. In general, this means you should borrow up to the maximum federal direct student loan amount that you need and then use your cash for any expenses above and beyond that amount until it runs out. The second principle is to use your cash earlier in your education to avoid the accumulation of interest during medical school. Sometimes these two principles conflict a bit, but if you keep them both in mind when deciding how to use your cash, you will choose a reasonable course. The main goal is to start your residency (or career, if you are a dentist going straight into practice) with all of your cash spent, with the minimum amount of loans, and with the most attractive loan terms possible.

If you have retirement account money in an Individual Retirement Arrangement (IRA), Roth IRA, 401(k), or similar account, I generally advise against tapping that to pay for your education. Since that money is both tax-protected and asset-protected, it is best to leave it compounding for your retirement. Nevertheless, you should be aware that if you do choose to use that money for your education, there are some special rules that apply, and they are a bit complicated. You can always withdraw as much as you want from a retirement account. However, if you withdraw money from the account prior to age 59½, you will owe a 10% penalty on the withdrawal, in addition to the taxes that would be due on withdrawals from a tax-deferred account. College or professional school costs are an exception to that 10% penalty, at least up to the amount of the legitimate educational expenses.

This exception only applies to an IRA, not a 401(k). So if you do choose to tap this source of funds for schooling, be sure to rollover your 401(k) to an IRA first. A Roth IRA is a tax-free account, but generally only for retirement. If you withdraw it for education, you may owe taxes on any earnings withdrawn. However, the account allows you to withdraw the principal first, which comes out tax-free. If you withdraw all of the principal and then start withdrawing the earnings, the earnings can also come out tax-free if used for education, but only if it has been at least five tax years since you first contributed to an IRA—a barrier that will exclude many medical and dental students in their first year of school but becomes lower and lower as they progress through school.

Withdrawing IRA Money to Use for Education		
Asset	Taxes Due?	Penalty Due?
Traditional IRA Principal	Yes	No
Traditional IRA Earnings	Yes	No
ROTH IRA Principal	No	No
ROTH IRA Earnings in Account <5 Years Old	Yes	Yes
ROTH IRA Earnings in Account >5 Years Old	No	No
401(k) Principal	Yes	Yes
ROTH 401(k) Principal	Yes	Yes

In case you are wondering, no, you cannot contribute student loan money into retirement accounts like IRAs; only earned income can go into retirement accounts. If you, like me when I was in medical school, have no idea what any of the terms in the last few paragraphs mean, stay tuned, we will get to them in the financial literacy section later in the book.

GET A DISCOUNT

There are some regional and medical school specific programs that allow you to pay resident tuition despite coming from out of state. Be sure to inquire about these before and even after you enroll in school. An example is the WWAMI (Washington, Wyoming, Alaska, Montana, Idaho) program, which allows students from those states to pay in-state tuition at The University of Washington. Another is the WICHE (Western Interstate Commission for Higher Education) program, which has similar features but includes far more Western states. My medical school, the University of Utah, by contract reserved a certain number of its seats for Idaho residents and allowed them to pay in-state tuition. There are likely similar agreements at other schools across the country. Read the fine print, as you are sometimes required to return to your home state to practice afterward.

MD/PHD PROGRAMS

There are numerous MD/PhD programs across the country. Several students in each class are generally enrolled, at least at medical schools associated with a large research institution. These students not only have their medical school tuition waived, but also often receive a stipend. By living frugally, it is entirely possible for these students to complete their education completely debt-free. The catch, of course, is that their education will take much longer than that of the "pure" medical students they start with. In general, they attend the first two years of medical school, then work on a PhD for 3–6 years, and then complete the last two years of medical school. The real cost of paying for medical school this way is the opportunity cost of not working as a physician for those 3–6 years while you are working on a PhD. That amount is likely to be $500,000 to a million dollars or even more, even after accounting for the PhD stipend and taxes.

Thus, this is not a financially savvy way to pay for medical school unless you really want to get a PhD. On average, these programs cut 2–3 years off the time required to get both an MD and a PhD and eliminate MD tuition. So you are far better off doing a combined MD/PhD than separate programs. It can be difficult to know what you want to do with your life and career when you are applying to medical school at age 21 or 22. Contracting with an MD/PhD program is a big commitment and should be taken very seriously. As high as 34% of MD/PhD matriculants drop out of the MD/PhD program. Most of those (86%) who drop out simply finish medical school and obtain their MD.[15] If you are considering quitting, read the contract. In general, the contract states you will need to pay back something like ⅔ of the stipend plus the first two years of medical school tuition. However, in practice, few students actually pay anything back, especially if they completed at least two years of graduate school. MD/PhD graduates generally become physician scientists at academic medical centers, a position that will usually qualify them for the Public Service Loan Forgiveness (PSLF) program anyway, so the main financial benefit of the program (waived medical school tuition) is not nearly as significant as you might expect in the long run. You can learn more about the PSLF program here:

Blog Post: Public Service Loan Forgiveness
www.whitecoatinvestor.com/public-service-loan-forgiveness/

MILITARY HEALTH PROFESSIONS SCHOLARSHIP PROGRAM

Another contract that is frequently used to pay for medical and dental school is the military Health Professions Scholarship Program (HPSP), the method I used to pay for my schooling. In my opinion, this program is misnamed as a scholarship. It is not a scholarship in the way the word is typically used; it is a contract. The military pays your tuition, fees, and required expenses as well as a taxable living stipend of about $2,200 per month in 2020. In exchange for this generous benefit, you will owe the military a year of active duty service as an attending for each year you received the scholarship. In addition, you will need to go through the military residency match process. Military physicians generally find they are paid less than they would be in civilian medicine, although this difference is much less significant for a primary care physician than a surgical subspecialist. In addition, the military will dictate the base you work on when not deployed to a war zone, when, where and for how long you will be deployed to war zones, your working hours, your co-workers, your dress (generally a military uniform), and many other aspects of professional and personal life.

Perhaps the biggest risk is the military match. The number of slots in a given specialty each year is determined by the military, no matter how many students entering the match wish to train in that specialty. This frequently results in a mismatch of the desires of the students with the needs of the military for a given specialty. In these situations, some students are not permitted to match into their chosen specialty. Instead, they are placed into an internship of some type (transitional, internal medicine, or surgery) and then, with only one year of post-graduate training, become some type of a general medical officer for the next two years. At that point they may be able to match into their chosen specialty, but failure to match a second time could mean another two years as a general medical officer. In addition, residency training in the military comes with its own commitment. Each year of residency training (after the first "intern" year) carries one year of payback requirement. However, your medical school commitment and your residency commitment run concurrently, so it is not usually a big deal if you match straight into your specialty. If you do not match for four years afterward, you may end up being committed to four years of medical school, a year of internship, four years as a general medical officer, four more years of residency training, and then four more years as a military physician. This is a risk that must be weighed when accepting an HPSP scholarship for medical school.

From a financial perspective, the more expensive the medical school and the lower the pay in your chosen specialty, the better off you will be financially for taking an HPSP scholarship. However, many doctors find the finances to be about the same either way—you just get more money upfront from the military and less money later. Thus, the primary factor in determining whether to pay for medical school using the HPSP scholarship should be whether or not you want to be a military physician, at least for the first part of your career. If you do, the HPSP is one of the best ways to pay for it. If you do not have a career goal to be a military physician, steer clear. You will likely endure significant misery if you sign up primarily to pay for school.

The dental HPSP program is a more attractive deal than the medical HPSP program because dental schools generally cost more, dentists generally earn less in the civilian world, and there is minimal concern about the military match. A new requirement in 2019, however, is that all graduating dentists must apply for a one-year general dentistry residency and complete it if accepted. This requirement will obviously lengthen the total time period you spend on active duty.

Military service seems a lot more exciting at 22 when you sign the contract than it might at 32, when it finally comes time to be deployed. At 22, you are likely single. At 32, you may have already started a family or be wanting to. While maternity and paternity leave has become more generous over the years, you still have to return to duty eventually. Just recognize that for many doctors the time they finally become a valuable, deployable asset to the military precisely overlaps with the time they want to start a family.

I know the paragraphs above paint military service and this scholarship in particular in an unfavorable light. However, I do not feel that hiding the facts about how the program works does anybody, including the military, any favors. I had a lot of wonderful experiences being in the military and there are a lot of wonderful aspects of a military practice and serving your country. However, given the frequent changes in military service, it would behoove any potential HPSP applicant, especially one without any prior active duty experience, to speak personally with several current active duty physicians (including at least one who is unhappy with the decision to join) prior to accepting the scholarship.

UNIFORMED SERVICES UNIVERSITY OF THE HEALTH SCIENCES

Another option for paying for medical school is to attend the military medical school, the Uniformed Services University of the Health Sciences (USUHS). While the commitment for this program is much higher (seven years instead of four) than the HPSP program, it pays a fair amount more, providing its students a regular 2nd lieutenant (or ensign) paycheck and allowances during those four years, approximately $60,000–$70,000 per year. All tuition and fees are covered as well. For those anticipating a longer military career, financially-speaking this is the best way to pay for medical school. Those considering this option should weigh the quality of education received against the other schools they were accepted to. Expect to do your third- and fourth-year rotations at multiple bases across the country mostly taking care of a relatively healthy population, although you may be able to do some of your rotations in civilian hospitals.

FINANCIAL ASSISTANCE PROGRAM

The military Financial Assistance Program (FAP) is a program designed for medical and dental residents. As a resident, you receive an annual grant of $45,000 (to put toward student loans) plus the same taxable monthly stipend an HPSP student would receive. Any required fees, books, equipment, and tuition is also covered. The primary benefit of this program over the HPSP program is that there is no requirement to go through the military match. The downside is that if you attended an expensive school, that $45,000 per year may not pay off your loans entirely. The commitment is two years on active duty for your first year of participation, plus one additional year for each year after that. You can combine the HPSP and FAP program, but the service commitments do not run concurrently.

NATIONAL GUARD

The National Guard also needs physicians and has several programs to encourage students, residents, and attending physicians to join. The student program is called the Medical and Dental Student Stipend Program (MDSSP). It pays $2,270 per month. For each year you receive this stipend, you will owe the Guard two years of service. Guard service includes two days a month, two weeks a year, and occasional 90-day deployments.

Following medical school, you would typically then enroll in the Specialized Training Assistance Program (STRAP). Once more, you receive a monthly stipend of $2,270 per month, incurring an obligation of two years of guard duty for each year of stipend receipt. Of note, each year in the STRAP program counts for a year of payback from the MDSSP program. So if you did four years of medical school, you would incur an eight-year service commitment. If that were followed by a three-year residency, you would pay off three of those eight years, while incurring a six-year commitment. So after residency, you would owe 8 + 6 - 3 = 11 years in the Guard.

The Guard is not interested in physicians of every specialty. Their current list of desired specialists includes:

> Cardiology
>
> Emergency Medicine
>
> Endocrinology
>
> Family Practice
>
> Gastroenterology
>
> General Surgery
>
> Infectious Disease
>
> Internal Medicine
>
> Medical Oncology/Hematology
>
> Nephrology
>
> OB/GYN
>
> Orthopedic Surgery
>
> Preventive Medicine
>
> Pulmonology
>
> Rheumatology

Notice the lack of pediatric and most surgical specialties.

Once you become at least a third-year resident (or practicing dentist), you are eligible for another National Guard program, called the Health Professions Loan Repayment Program (HPLRP), which will pay $40,000 per year toward your student loans until the loans are gone, up to a maximum of seven years and $250,000. (Note that during the last year you would only qualify for $10,000.) This is in exchange for a "year-for-year" service commitment, up to 7 years, which is in addition to your other commitments. Thus a student who took MDSSP, STRAP in a four-year residency program, and a full seven-year HPLRP, would have an $8 + 8 - 4 + 7 = 19$-year service commitment in the Guard. There are other bonus payments available including the Officer Accession Bonus and a retention bonus.

Similar to the MD/PhD and HPSP programs, this is a great program if you want to serve in the Guard anyway, but involves too large of a commitment to do just for the money to pay for medical school. While the commitment is much longer than that incurred for the HPSP scholarship, it is far less onerous given the relative ease of Guard service, the ability to simply go through the civilian residency match, and the ability to still have a civilian career.

NATIONAL HEALTH SERVICE CORPS

The National Health Service Corps (NHSC) has a "scholarship" program for physicians, dentists, and other professions similar to the HPSP program, but without the deployments. US citizens and nationals are eligible, even if attending many international medical schools, as long as they are going into primary care or dentistry. It covers tuition, pays fees, and provides the same taxable monthly stipend that HPSP students get—$1,419 in 2020.

The commitment, however, is two years of service for each year of scholarship received. This service is performed in a designated Health Professional Shortage Area. These include specific geographic areas, specific populations, or specific facilities, such as community health centers, correctional facilities, state mental hospitals, and some Indian health facilities. Like with the military contracts, this is a great option for someone who wishes to have a career, or at least spend a few years, working with an underserved community.

In addition to the scholarship program, there is a loan repayment program for doctors of eligible specialties, including dentistry. The amount of money you receive depends on how needy the community is and whether you commit to full-time or half-time practice, but can be as much as a non-taxable $50,000 total for a two-year full-time commitment. Obviously, this is much less money than you would receive for the same commitment under the scholarship program.

INDIAN HEALTH SERVICES

The Indian Health Services (IHS) also has a "scholarship" (read "contract") program. In order to receive this, you must be a member of a federally recognized American Indian Tribe or Alaska Native village. It provides a taxable monthly living stipend of at least $1,500 and covers all tuition and fees. The commitment is one year of service for each year of scholarship receipt, with a minimum of two years. You must serve at a designated Indian Health Service facility or other practice where at least 75% of the practice population consists of Native Americans.

STATE REPAYMENT PROGRAMS

Many states have programs where they will repay part or all of your medical school loans in exchange for a service commitment of at least two years. These are generally primary care positions in rural or underserved communities. Unlike most military, NHSC, and IHS qualifying jobs, these jobs often provide a higher salary in addition to the loan repayment. These loan repayments may be taxable.

EMPLOYER LOAN REPAYMENT PROGRAMS

Many private employers also offer loan repayment programs. This benefit is generally taxable, although recent laws have made at least a small portion tax-free to the employee while still being deductible to the employer. Be aware that for the most part employers look at this sort of a benefit as something that is given in lieu of a higher salary, rather than in addition to a higher salary, but it does provide an additional point of negotiation when taking that first job out of training.

PUBLIC SERVICE LOAN FORGIVENESS

After simply paying off your student loans yourself, the Public Service Loan Forgiveness (PSLF) program is likely the next most popular method of paying for medical school. Under this program, a student who makes 120 on-time, monthly payments on qualifying federal direct loans through a qualifying program such as the federal Income-Driven Repayment (IDR) programs while working full-time for a qualifying federal, state, or non-profit 501(c)(3) employer, will have any remaining debt forgiven tax-free. This program officially started in 2007, making the first cohort of eligible borrowers qualify to receive forgiveness in 2017. However, for various reasons, very few doctors will receive any forgiveness prior to 2021–2023, at which point more and more borrowers each year will qualify. The typical person for whom this program will work well has a large federal student loan burden, spent a long time in residency and fellowship, and was already planning on an academic career, at least for the first few years out of training. Thanks to the IDR programs, payments during residency and fellowship can be as low as $0 per month, but they still count toward the 120 payments. Thus, a doctor who spends three years in residency and three more in fellowship, may only make substantial payments for three or four years before the remainder, potentially hundreds of thousands of dollars, is forgiven tax-free.

If this is your planned method to pay for medical school, keep careful records of every qualifying payment made and your annual employer certification forms. Be sure to fill out the application correctly. In the first year of possible forgiveness (2017), 99% of applicants were rejected. While the majority did not qualify for various reasons (ineligible loans, ineligible loan program, ineligible employer, etc.), a substantial minority simply did not fill out the application correctly. Another substantial minority ran into a problem where the loan servicing company undercounted their qualifying payments, thus the need to keep your own careful records. It is not advantageous to the government or the loan servicing company representing the government to grant you forgiveness, so expect a bit of a fight to get it. Some have found they had to employ a lawyer or a student loan specialist in order to receive the forgiveness they deserved.

IDR FORGIVENESS

The Income-Driven Repayment (IDR) programs have their own forgiveness programs that do not require you to work full-time for a 501(c)(3) or government employer. However, these programs have two substantial downsides. The first is that they require you to make 20–25 years of payments, rather than just 10. Most doctors will have paid off their loans completely by that time, even making minimum payments. The second downside is that the forgiveness is taxable at your ordinary income tax rates in the year that it is received. For those with a substantial debt-to-income ratio, this "tax bomb" may be larger than your loans were originally! These downsides make these programs unattractive to the vast majority of borrowers, but there are a few people for whom they could make sense—primarily those with very high debt-to-income ratios and an inability to find or unwillingness to take a job that qualifies for PSLF.

TAKE OUT STUDENT LOANS AND PAY THEM BACK

Approximately 27% of medical students graduate debt-free, although many of those have an HPSP, NHSC, or similar contract. The remaining 73% borrowed at least some money. While a fair number will have their loans forgiven or paid off by an employer, the vast majority will simply have to pay off their student loans themselves. The good news is that this is still very doable, but only for those doctors who can control their spending after they come out of their training period. Too many doctors grow right into their newfound high income; but if they can simply delay doing that for 2–5 years, living the same lifestyle they had as a medical resident or dental student, almost all of them can be debt-free within half a decade of completion.

With frugal living, it is entirely possible for doctors to dedicate $5,000, $8,000, $10,000, or even $15,000 per month toward their student loans. Paying $10,000 per month toward your student loans will wipe out even a half-million-dollar debt in just five years. Since the average debt is about half that, many doctors can be debt-free in less time than it would take to pay off an HPSP or NHSC commitment or complete a PhD. But they must be financially disciplined enough to actually do it. I call this philosophy "Live like a Resident." If you (and your partner, if any) will commit now to do so, you can be assured that you will have a financially awesome life (eventually) and can spend a lot less time worrying about money during school. This truly is the secret to becoming a rich doctor down the road. Refinancing those student loans can help you pay them back because a larger portion of your payment will then go toward principal instead of interest. You can see the best deals for refinancing your student loans here:

Resource: Refinance Medical School Loans & Consolidation Guide
www.whitecoatinvestor.com/student-loan-refinancing/

A FEW WORDS ABOUT FAMILY LOANS

Sometimes a family member would like to help you out with the cost of medical school. If that "help" is a gift, I suggest you tell them "thank you," cash the check, and go on your merry way. If that help is a loan, you need to "look that gift horse in the mouth." While a family member will often cut you a better deal than the government in the form of lower fees, less hassle, and a lower interest rate, Thanksgiving dinner does not taste the same when you owe money to someone else at the table.

The loan may also be illegal. If you accept a loan from a family member, put together a basic promissory note outlining how interest will be calculated, how payments will be calculated, when payments will be due, whether or not you can pre-pay the loan, and under what circumstances the loan may be forgiven. The IRS requires family loans to charge a minimum interest rate that varies each year and by the length of the loan. In June of 2020 as I write this chapter, with interest rates at all-time lows, a short-term loan (< 3 years) can charge as little as 0.18%. Even a long-term loan (>9 years) only has to charge 1.01%. However, 20 years ago those rates were over 6%.

Any interest that is not charged is considered a gift for tax purposes. That is not a problem for amounts less than the $15,000 (in 2020) per year gift tax limits. Even forgiven interest above $15,000 per year may not be a big deal if the lender is far below the applicable federal and state estate tax exemption limits, but a gift tax return will need to be filed. Family lenders who do not live in the US may care less about what the IRS thinks of their loan, but they should look into their own tax laws to see if similar rules exist.

Sometimes parents borrow money for their child's education, either through the federal government's Parent PLUS Loans, via a private student loan lender, through a home equity line of credit (HELOC), or using credit cards. I think this is generally a bad idea. In my opinion, if anyone is going to borrow money, it should be the student. That will allow them to have "skin in the game," take advantage of any federal forgiveness or income-driven repayment programs, and be able to discharge the debt easily in the event of death or permanent disability.

In the event that you do borrow money from family, be sure to protect them by getting adequate term life and disability insurance as soon as feasible. You do not want them to be left holding the bag if something happens to you.

I would also give serious consideration to the financial stability of the family member before accepting a loan, or even a gift, from them. As a practicing doctor willing to manage your money properly, you are going to have the ability to pay for your education eventually. But that does not mean that a loan to you is the family member's best use for their money. You do not necessarily want a family member to give you money that should have gone toward their retirement or mortgage, and then find out you will be supporting them later in life! Every family and culture are different in this regard, and this should be navigated according to your personal situation. As a general rule, retirement should be a much higher priority for parents than the schooling of their children. Parental financial independence is one of the greatest gifts that can be given to children. Taking money from your financially precarious parents now may mean they are living in your basement later!

Medical and dental school are expensive. Although a few schools have implemented free tuition for some or all of their students, the likely future for most involves a higher and higher price each year for this education. If you will be smart about how you pay for it, you will pave your pathway to financial stability and freedom down the road.

MAIN IDEAS

- Pay for your schooling with cash if you and your family can afford to do so.

- About ¾ of students borrow to pay for school.

- Scholarships, loan repayment/forgiveness programs, and unique opportunities are available to help decrease the cost of school.

- Beware of "scholarship programs" that are really employment contracts. Understand what you are signing.

ADDITIONAL RESOURCES

- **Blog Post:** Don't Give Up on PSLF Loan Forgiveness *www.whitecoatinvestor.com/dont-give-up-pslf/*

- **Blog Post:** Should I Join the Military to Pay for Medical School? *www.whitecoatinvestor.com/personal-finance/should-i-join-the-military-to-pay-for-medical-school/*

- **Blog Post:** The Health Professions Scholarship Program *www.whitecoatinvestor.com/the-health-professions-scholarship-program-hpsp-scholarship/*

- **Website:** Army Medicine: Health Professions Scholarship Program *www.goarmy.com/amedd/education/hpsp.html*

- **Blog Post:** Army National Guard Physicians *www.whitecoatinvestor.com/army-national-guard-physicians/*

- **Blog Post:** NHSC—Loan Repayment or Scholarship? *www.whitecoatinvestor.com/nhsc-loan-repayment-or-scholarship/*

- **Blog Post:** How to Pay Off Medical School Loans in Less than 2 Years *www.whitecoatinvestor.com/how-to-pay-off-medical-school-loans-in-less-than-2-years/*

- **Blog Post:** How Fast Can You Get Out of Debt? *www.whitecoatinvestor.com/how-fast-can-you-get-out-of-debt/*

CHAPTER FIVE

WHY YOU SHOULD BE A THRIFTY STUDENT

Thrift is a critical financial principle for just about anyone, but it is particularly important for someone who is going to spend most of their 20s in school. Living within your means, or even below your means, allows interest to work for you instead of against you. When you are paying for school with debt, by definition you are living above your means. Each month you sink further and further into debt.

Minimizing how far you go into debt is key to your finances. After you select a school to attend, the main way you can do this is by spending as little as possible. If you borrow money at 8% as an MS1 and the interest compounds through four years of medical school, three years of residency, three years of fellowship, and then is paid off over 20 years, that first $100 you borrowed will have 8% compound interest working on it for three full decades. At 8%, that $100 will have grown to over $1,000. In essence, whatever you paid for with those first borrowed dollars was really 10 times the sticker price. A more realistic scenario perhaps involves a period of 15 years and an average interest rate of 6% for your average borrowed dollar. But even there, you are paying 2 ½ times the sticker price for whatever you bought with that borrowed money. Every computer, every meal out, every car, every bus pass really costs 2.5X what you think you are paying for it when you are buying it on debt as a medical student.

It gets even worse when you realize how our tax code works. Our tax code is quite progressive and the money you use to pay that money back later as an attending physician or dentist may have been subject to a marginal tax

45

rate of 30%, 40%, or more when you include state income tax. After taking that into account, you have to earn 3.5X (or more) to pay for your in-school purchases.

Those numbers demonstrate just how important it is to keep your debt burden down. Yes, you will probably have a high income down the road. But if you match it with a very high debt burden, a great deal of that income (and your hard work) will go toward servicing the debt. Make smart and thrifty spending choices now and your future self will thank you later.

One of the most expensive things you can do as a student is take an extra year to graduate. Whether a gap year, a research year, an MPH or similar degree, time to care for a family member, or just additional time to complete your studies, it all has the same financial impact. You will have to cover your living expenses and you might have to pay additional tuition. But the most significant expense is the future opportunity cost of earning a doctor salary for one fewer year during your career. Looking at it that way, it is a very expensive year. So you need to be very sure that the benefits outweigh the costs in your individual situation. Most doctors can still make plenty of money to pay off their loans and become multimillionaires before retirement even with a gap year, but to pretend there is no financial impact would be silly.

Since most medical students do not take out private loans (usually at higher interest rates) until they have maximized their use of direct federal loans (usually at lower interest rates), keeping your spending down can help you maintain a lower ratio of private to federal loans and save interest along the way. While many students cannot completely avoid using private loans, you are almost always better off with less of them! Federal loans are also the only ones eligible for the Income-Driven Repayment (IDR) and Public Service Loan Forgiveness programs (PSLF) we will discuss later.

Another reason to live frugally in medical school is well-grounded in the behavioral finance sphere. It is psychologically much easier to increase your standard of living than to decrease it. This tendency we all have to grow into our income is called lifestyle inflation or the hedonic treadmill. Despite spending more, we do not permanently increase our happiness. It also turns out that many small increases in spending actually bring more happiness than one large increase in spending. If you live frugally as a student, the modest upgrades in lifestyle in residency will feel like splurges and bring on more enjoyment. Alternatively, if you live large in school trying to keep up with wealthy or financially illiterate peers, then it may feel like you are going backwards if you have to cut back in residency (especially if your residency is in a high-cost-of-living city).

One of the initial reviewers of this book said:

> "At this point in the book I was noting all the mistakes I made as a student (I currently have $600,000 in student loan debt). If I could go back in time I would beat myself until I had hematuria and yell that I should get a cheaper education and be thrifty at every opportunity. Please encourage students not to be passive about what they are reading in this chapter."

I am not sure there is anything I can say that will be more powerful than that to encourage you to spend less during school. Previous generations had a mantra, "Use it up, wear it out, make it do, or do without."

Before buying anything, consider ways you can delay the purchase, buy less of it, pay less for it, or avoid buying it at all. Thrifty living as a medical or dental student not only helps you build the financial "muscles" that will later serve you well, but it also helps you to minimize the size of the debt mountain you must climb upon completing your training.

MAIN IDEAS

- Living on borrowed money is really expensive.

- Lessons in thrift and frugality learned as a student will build the "financial muscles" that will make you successful later.

ADDITIONAL RESOURCES

- **Blog Post:** The Frugal Physician: Self-Serving or Self-Denying?
  www.physicianonfire.com/the-frugal-physician-self-serving-or-self-denial/

- **Blog Post:** The Frugal Physician: 5 Steps to Becoming Debt-Free
  www.whitecoatinvestor.com/frugal-physician-5-steps-debt-free/

- **Blog Post:** How to Get Rich Driving a $5,000 Car
  www.whitecoatinvestor.com/how-to-get-rich-by-driving-a-5000-car/

CHAPTER SIX

HOW TO LIVE ON LOANS

I have read dozens of financial books and thousands of blog posts. I do not recall ever seeing a single instance where a writer has explained how to live on borrowed money. It simply is not a subject that is covered. Yet the vast majority of the doctors in our country have done this for four or more years of their lives. It is a bit ironic that I am the doctor to write this chapter since I did not actually live on loans during medical school, but someone has to do it and I have certainly spoken with enough people doing it that I think I can share a few words of wisdom about it.

The main goal I have with this chapter is to eliminate the guilt you may feel from living on loans. While my secondary goal is to help you minimize how much debt you leave medical or dental school with, that is no reason to spend four years beating yourself up about the method you have chosen to use to pay for your education. Once you have made the decision to pay for your schooling with borrowed money, and committed to paying that debt off on a short timeline after finishing training by "living like a resident" until it is gone, let it go. Seriously. Quit stressing about it. Lying awake at night worrying about it is not only counter-productive but entirely unjustified. Concentrate on your studies and become the best doctor you can. So long as you become a practicing physician or dentist and live like a resident until the debt is gone, you will be able to pay off this debt.

Part of the guilt comes from our society. In general, those who avoid debt are considered virtuous while those who are mired in debt are considered undisciplined spendthrifts. Financial shows on the radio bring on callers to scream "I'm debt-free!" with regularity. I have news for you. Most people will never be able to save up $200,000–$400,000 prior to starting school, nor will they be able to cash flow that sort of a sum. I would love to see that change, but I also recognize it is unlikely to happen any time soon.

We have to play the game with the cards we are dealt. If we actually want to have enough doctors in this country, we either accept that many doctors will have to borrow significant sums of money, or we only allow the children of the wealthy to go to medical or dental school. Most credit card, auto, and other consumer debt does not dramatically increase your ability to earn money down the road. But your student loans do. We do not think it is morally wrong for a business to borrow some money to open a second store, and it is not wrong to borrow a reasonable amount of money to pay for a degree that will provide a great return on the investment.

Another part of the guilt comes from ourselves. We see over ¼ of our classmates graduating without any debt at all. However, we fail to realize that those classmates are not like us. Maybe they have a physician, attorney, or business owner spouse. Perhaps they had a $300,000 529 account waiting for them when they graduated from high school. More likely, they have taken on a different type of debt, like I did, and owe time to the military, National Guard, NHSC, or IHS. Forget about it. You have a plan. It is a reasonable plan. It will work. Now execute it and quit worrying about what other people are doing or thinking.

HOW TO MINIMIZE YOUR LOANS

Now that we have that rant out of the way, we should talk about how to minimize how much you owe at the end of medical school. While I do not want you to feel guilty about having debt, it would be a disservice to tell you that there is no difference in your future financial life if you come out owing $400,000 instead of $250,000. This is not Monopoly money that you are signing for each semester. It really will have to be paid back, and if you do not pay it off quickly, by the time you do pay it off everything you are purchasing now with borrowed money may really "cost" 3–5 times as much as you think you are paying for it. Living frugally during school really will help reduce the burden and reduce the amount of time you have to live like a resident in order to pay it off. Living on $50,000 a year while earning $300,000 a year is not pleasant, requires discipline, and is going to be harder than you think. Do not extend that time period any longer than you have to.

HOW TO LIVE ON LOANS

One factor that works to your advantage when you are trying to live frugally during school is that everybody around you is broke too. Once you graduate, family, friends, neighbors, and patients will all expect you to live like a doctor. But for now, everybody understands you are a student and have no money. So it is much easier to live like it. You can turn down invitations to eat out, you can drive an older economy car (or better yet walk, bike, or ride the bus), and live in a dumpy apartment. You do not need the latest fashions, the most organic food, or the fanciest vacations. Find free things to do that you love.

If you are single, get some roommates. Aside from tuition, rent is likely your largest expense. Cut it in half, or by 75%, by picking up a roommate or three. If you have a partner, you may not want roommates, but there is still an economy of scale there. If you have kids, buy your baby gear off of Craigslist for 10% of the cost instead of brand new. Furniture rapidly depreciates. Used couches and tables are routinely sold for pennies on the dollar. Maybe you are grossed out buying a used mattress. Fine. But you can certainly get a used bed frame and box spring. Or no bedframe at all. We did not spend a lot of money in medical school, but I still look back on it as four of the best years of our lives. You are not what you spend.

Another way to reduce your loan burden is to wait until you actually need the money before you borrow it. Most students take out enough money to cover the entire school year in August. That interest starts ticking from the moment you sign for the loan. There is no reason to do that. If you need more money later, you can usually get it within a couple of weeks. So wait until you need the loan money before you take it out. Loans taken out in March instead of August saved 8 months of interest. At 7% on $20,000, that is $933. That could cover an entire month of rent.

This idea can even be carried to an extreme. Credit cards will often offer a 0% introductory deal that lasts for 12–15 months. This allows you to put your living expenses on a credit card and then just before the interest starts accumulating, to take out that student loan and pay off the credit card with it. Obviously, you need reasonably high credit card limits in order to do this, so it may not be an option for many traditional students with no prior career or significant credit history. Be aware that studies show that we tend to spend more money when we use credit cards for our spending. You do not have to spend much more to eliminate the benefit you are trying to achieve here. You really need to know yourself before you attempt a stunt like that.

Travel hacking is one way that some savvy students still manage to indulge their love of travel while living on a bare-bones budget in school. Travel hacking involves working within the existing rules set up by airlines, credit cards, and hotels, and using them to your advantage to earn free travel including flights, lodging, and other upgrades. Be careful not to get burned using credit cards, but there are entire books, blogs, and forums dedicated to this art.

Family gift money, such as that often given for birthdays or Christmas can also be used strategically to lower your indebtedness.

BUDGETING BORROWED MONEY

It probably feels a little funny to live on a budget when there is no real income actually coming in. It also feels weird to limit yourself when you know you can just go back to the financial aid office, sign your name, and get another few thousand dollars any time you want. However, these four years of school are the ideal time to learn how to live on a budget. Learn to estimate your expenses in advance. Be as exact as you can, but recognize that "things will come up," so add a little bit extra into the budget so you can take care of them and do not constantly feel deprived or guilty for busting the budget. If your budget says you need $2,000 a month, then borrow $2,000 a month. When the $2,000 runs out, stop spending, just like it was a real income.

If you have never budgeted before, it can be intimidating to do the first time. The key is to find a method that works for you. It can be done most simply by using paper and pencil and keeping cash in envelopes. Others prefer to spend using only a debit card and/or checks. In addition, many people prefer to use technological aids to assist them in the process. A simple spreadsheet on Google Sheets or Microsoft Excel can do the math for you and allow you to copy and paste from month to month. Phone or computer apps such as You Need a Budget®, Mint®, or EveryDollar® help many people, especially when they have to coordinate spending between two people. No matter how you choose to do it, the key is to assign dollar amounts to various categories of spending and then stop spending in that category when you run out of money. The only exception is when you reduce spending in another category to make up for it. A "zero-based" budget tries to "give every dollar a name." So at the beginning of the month, you know exactly where your money is going to go. Budgeting categories may include:

Rent

Utilities

Groceries

Gasoline

Insurance

Schooling Costs

Clothing

Car Repairs

Health Care

Entertainment

I considered putting together a sample budget for you with actual dollar figures in each line. The problem with doing so is that budgets are so different from one person or family to another. This is not a bad thing, after all, a budget reflects your own personal values. The idea is to align your spending with what you truly care about. The problem is that any sample budget I gave you would just reflect my values. You would look at it and think I was crazy for spending so much on one thing and stupid for putting so little into another category. A married medical student might have a $2,000 rent payment while a single medical student with multiple roommates might only budget $300 in rent! Or even live rent-free with parents. So, unfortunately, I must leave this task to you.

Most budgeters use categories called "sinking funds" for expenses that do not occur every month. Health care expenses may be a good example. Perhaps some months you spend nothing but once or twice a year have a big bill. With a sinking fund, you are putting money into that category every month so that it is there when the big bill comes due. I think this is a good idea when living on a real income, but you may or may not wish to do it while living on loans. You may wish to simply deal with infrequent but large expenses by taking out additional loans just in time to cover those expenses. This may help minimize interest paid.

Many students and their partners see luxuries, vacations, and expensive wants as normal expectations because everyone else does it. Realizing these expectations are contrived, are unnecessary, and do not bring true happiness can free you from the (usually unconscious) desire to "keep up with the Joneses."

Remember that most successful budgeters do not have immediate success. It takes a few months to figure out how to do this. Give yourself a little grace and just try to get better at it each month. You will become better at foreseeing and estimating your future living expenses. You will become more disciplined at telling yourself (and your friends, and your partner), "No, I cannot afford that right now." These skills you learn during school are like financial muscles. As you exercise them, they will become stronger. They will allow you to live within your means and even begin to save as a resident. And if you apply them to your attending income, watch out! You will become wealthy faster than you ever imagined. This will give you the freedom to do whatever you want with your life, to help those around you, and to enjoy what this world has to offer along the way.

YOU MAY QUALIFY FOR MANY GOVERNMENT PROGRAMS

Most government assistance programs are designed for people with little in assets and little in income, but few of them ask if you are in school learning something that will pay you hundreds of thousands of dollars down the road. Thus, most medical and dental students, especially those with families, qualify for services such as Medicaid, food stamps, cash assistance, housing assistance, and health insurance subsidies. If you have some earned income, you likely qualify for the Earned Income Tax Credit, another social redistribution program embedded in the tax code. There is a federal tax credit for savers that a few medical student couples and new interns can take advantage of. You might even find yourself in a position where a federal or state down payment assistance program can help you. While some students feel morally wrong about taking money from the government, recognize that the best use of these programs is to make it so people no longer qualify for the programs by helping them obtain education, training, and jobs that will make them more money! Besides, I assure you that during your career you will pay all of those benefits back many times in the form of high tax bills! Do not cheat or lie on the applications, but if you qualify, you qualify.

YOU CAN WORK DURING MEDICAL SCHOOL

Some medical and dental schools prohibit you from working. But many do not. Instead, your ability to perform paid work is simply dependent on your academic workload and your ability to manage it. Now I am not saying you should try to hold down a full-time job while doing your OB/GYN rotation during your third year of school. As the Preacher said in Ecclesiastes, "There is...a time to plant and a time to pluck up that which is planted...a time to get and a time to lose."[16] Medical school, dental school, and residency are not times to earn as much money as you can, but anything you can earn will reduce how much you need to borrow to complete your education. For medical students, the summer between your first and second year is an obvious candidate for paid work. While other students are off gallivanting across Europe or doing research, you could take a paid job for a few months. Or better yet, find a paid job doing research!

The last half of the fourth year of medical school is another great candidate. The work can even be medically related. I used free time during my fourth year of school to take histories and do pre-operative exams for the local surgical center. The surgeons signed off on them but it saved them so much time they were glad to pay me $20 an hour (the equivalent of $36 per hour today) to do them. If you had a prior career, perhaps you can continue to do some p.r.n. (as needed) or consulting work there when your schedule allows. Maybe you could teach MCAT prep classes on Friday evenings and Saturdays during your first couple of years. Perhaps if you are a good test taker you can study for four weeks for USMLE Step 1 instead of eight weeks, leaving you a month to work. The test will soon be pass-fail anyway. Do not let paid work get in the way of your education, but let us not kid ourselves that any of us studied 80 hours a week every week of medical school. Maintain balance and moderation, but use that creativity of yours and you may be surprised how much income you can generate on the side.

Dental students may not have as many opportunities to work as medical students, but they are sure to have more evenings and weekends off. DoorDash, Lyft, and similar "gig economy" jobs that you can pick up and put down at your leisure can provide significant income.

Side gigs that you may not even think of as work can also bring in income. One early reviewer of this book found creative ways to earn money in medical school and residency that included AirBNB and tutoring. That income can be used to pay for essentials or perhaps a few little extras that help you stay sane during this trying period of life.

YOUR PARTNER CAN WORK DURING SCHOOL

One of the greatest sources of income possible during school is your partner's income. Even if your partner is not an attending physician or high-powered attorney, even a middle-class job goes a long way for a family suffering through medical or dental school. Sometimes if your spouse works for the university, they and their family members qualify for reduced or free tuition. 50% off medical school tuition might be the equivalent of a $30,000 a year raise! Even if your spouse's income only covers living expenses and you still have to borrow every dollar of tuition, that would still allow you to reduce your debt burden by a six-figure amount.

SCHOLARSHIPS EXIST

When I was a medical student, I was surprisingly naive about the existence of scholarships. While they are not nearly as prevalent as they are for undergraduate students, they do still exist. Find out about as many as you qualify for and apply for them. Your financial aid office can help. They know of a lot more scholarships than they announce to the entire school. Be the squeaky wheel so you find out about every one of them as early as possible. A few years ago, we started The White Coat Investor Scholarship (learn more at *www.whitecoatinvestor.com/scholarship*) that gives away tens of thousands of dollars in cash and prizes to deserving professional students. It allows us to give back to the community, promote financial literacy among students, and directly reduce the student loan burden for a few of them. Despite us sending information about it every year to every medical and dental school in the country, surprisingly few financial aid officers pass the information on to their students. I suspect that is the case for many scholarship opportunities.

Living on loans is the reality for almost three-quarters of medical and dental students. That is not going to change any time soon. While you should not feel guilty about this, do everything you can to minimize how much you borrow during school. Future "you" will be very grateful.

MAIN IDEAS

- If you will "live like a resident" for 2–5 years after school, you can pay off your student loans very quickly.

- If you have a plan to wipe out your debt quickly after school, you should not feel guilty about living on borrowed money during school.

- Budgeting is tricky on borrowed money, but it can and should be done.

- Look into government programs; they are designed for poor people like students.

- Look into opportunities to earn income, even during school, to reduce indebtedness.

ADDITIONAL RESOURCES

- **Blog Post:** The Right Way to Use Debt in Medical School
  www.whitecoatinvestor.com/medical-school-debt/

- **Blog Post:** Hitting a Net Worth of $0 as an Intern
  www.whitecoatinvestor.com/hitting-a-net-worth-of-0-as-an-intern/

- **Blog Post:** Live like a Resident
  www.whitecoatinvestor.com/live-like-a-resident/

CHAPTER SEVEN

THE ADVANTAGES OF BEING A NON-TRADITIONAL STUDENT

The angst among non-traditional students is palpable, and I never really understood why. I once saw a 25-year-old matriculant wondering if she was too old for medical school. I do not know that anyone has ever really defined traditional versus non-traditional, but the average age for starting medical and dental students is certainly higher than 22 years old, especially when so many people do a gap year or two for various reasons. The 2019 American Association of Medical Colleges (AAMC) Matriculating Student Questionnaire notes that 32% of matriculants are 20–22, 52% are 23–25, 10% are 26–28, and 6% are over 28.[17]

Personally, I took two years off from college to perform unpaid missionary service. I have no regrets whatsoever about doing so as those two years were incredibly formative in both my professional and personal life. I came home a better student and frankly, a less selfish, more mature person ready to embark on the career of service that defines medicine. The empathy, study skills, and communication skills I learned have made me a far better doctor. Learning Spanish, a language I still use during most of my shifts in the emergency department, did not hurt either.

However, the disadvantages of starting your professional education a little later in life are obvious. First, it is easy to forget what you learned as an undergraduate after a few years. Second, you are more likely to be balancing family obligations with your schooling. Third, there is opportunity cost. In this case, every year of your career that you are not earning an attending physician or doctor salary represents the loss of a low to mid six-figure amount. Obviously, there is more to life than money, but this opportunity cost can really add up if you spend 10 years of your career earning an average income instead of a doctor income.

There are advantages as well. Medical schools like students who have a bit more life experience and maturity. You are simply more likely to know what you want out of life. There are several financial advantages as well. You are more likely to have a spouse or partner that can contribute to the costs of your education. You are more likely to have paid off other debts, such as undergraduate student loans, auto loans, or credit card loans. You have more experience managing money. You may have some savings put away that can be used to pay for school. You may have already started to save for retirement or college. You may already have substantial home equity.

Do what you can to minimize your disadvantages and maximize your advantages. For example, you could avoid doing additional research years. Ensure you match the first time you apply by spending a little more time and effort to rotate, apply, and interview widely. Apply to a few more "safety programs." Be a little more skeptical of doing fellowships that do not increase your earning power. All of these changes will help to minimize the effects of your late start.

Use your partner's earnings and any savings you may have to minimize the amount of debt you take out. If you can keep your student loan burden below $100,000, you can be out of debt years sooner than the average student in your class. As mentioned in the "How to Pay for Professional School" chapter, use savings to avoid loans with poor terms and to delay the onset of the student loan interest clock.

Many non-traditional students have a small balance in retirement accounts at the time they enroll in medical school. You can tap a traditional IRA penalty-free (but not tax-free) to pay for educational expenses. Roth IRA principal can be accessed penalty-free and tax-free, and if you have had a Roth IRA for more than five tax years, you can even withdraw the earnings penalty-free (but not tax-free). However, I generally recommend against using your retirement accounts to pay for school. Retirement accounts are tax-protected and asset-protected, and you will soon find yourself as an attending physician wishing you had more space to invest inside retirement accounts. That tax-protection allows your money to grow faster.

THE ADVANTAGES OF BEING A NON-TRADITIONAL STUDENT

Savvy non-traditional matriculants use tax-deferred accounts preferentially prior to enrolling in school, then take advantage of the three calendar years during professional school when they have little to no taxable income to do Roth conversions. A Roth conversion is moving money from a tax-deferred (or traditional) retirement account to a tax-free (or Roth) account, and pre-paying the taxes on those dollars. However, during medical or dental school you are likely in the lowest tax bracket of your life. If you are single and have no other taxable income, you could convert over $12,000 per year without any tax cost at all and over $60,000 per year paying no more than 12% in federal taxes on any given dollar in the account. You can double those figures if you are married to a non-earner. Even if you had to pay for those conversions with borrowed money, it would still be a good idea. However, keep in mind when you sign for a federal student loan you are certifying that you are only using the money for true educational costs, not Roth conversions! (More information about Roth conversions can be found at *www.whitecoatinvestor.com/roth-conversions/.*)

If you have substantial home equity, you may wish to take out a home equity line of credit (HELOC) and use that equity to pay for part or all of school. Be sure to apply for that HELOC well before you quit your job and start medical school, of course. They probably will not give it to you if you have no income. You do not have to actually take any money out before quitting your job to start school, but you do need to have it established. The HELOC interest rate is likely to be lower than that of your student loans. Mortgage interest on up to $100,000 on these loans used to be tax-deductible no matter what you used the money for, but under current law, only the interest used to pay for acquisition or renovation of the home is deductible.

If you happen to have a taxable investing account or rental properties, use the income from these investments to pay for your schooling. In fact, I would give serious consideration to liquidating these investments to further reduce how much you borrow.

Non-traditional students can be real assets to their classmates and the profession, but there is a personal and financial cost to going back to school. Minimize it as much as you can and give serious consideration to doing Roth conversions of any retirement accounts from your prior employer(s).

MAIN IDEAS

- Being a non-traditional student has advantages.

- Try to minimize the main financial disadvantage of a non-traditional student (opportunity cost).

- Use any savings from a prior career wisely.

ADDITIONAL RESOURCES

- **Article:** Medical School Costs for Non-Traditional Students *students-residents.aamc.org/choosing-medical-career/ article/medical-school-costs-for-non-traditional- students/*

- **Blog Post:** 10 Tips for Non-Traditional Medical School Applicants *www.kevinmd.com/blog/2019/01/10-tips-for-non- traditional-medical-school-applicants.html*

CHAPTER EIGHT

HOW TO CHOOSE A SPECIALTY (PHYSICIANS)

Perhaps the most difficult choice you will need to make in medical school, and certainly the most important financial one, is what specialty you will practice the rest of your career. Unlike nurses or advanced practice clinicians like physician assistants and nurse practitioners, physicians cannot easily change from one specialty to the other with just a few weeks or months of on-the-job training. If you want to go practice another specialty, you will need to complete another 3–6 years of residency or fellowship training, and at most will receive just 6–12 months of "credit" from your previous residency training. This turns specialty selection into a high-stakes decision, and unfortunately a decision that must be made without all of the information you really need to make it.

Ideally, you will have made this decision by the summer between your third and fourth year of school. Unfortunately, at that point in your education you have only rotated through the major specialties (Internal Medicine, Pediatrics, General Surgery, OB/GYN, and Psychiatry) and perhaps 1–2 electives. There are currently 135 recognized specialties and subspecialties in the United States medical system. These include:

- Abdominal Radiology, Diagnostic Radiology
- Addiction Psychiatry, Psychiatry
- Adolescent Medicine, Pediatrics
- Adult Cardiothoracic Anesthesiology, Anesthesiology

- Adult Reconstructive Orthopedics, Orthopedic Surgery
- Advanced Heart Failure and Transplant Cardiology, Internal Medicine
- Allergy and Immunology
- Anatomic and Clinical Pathology
- Anesthesiology
- Biochemical Genetics, Medical Genetics
- Blood Banking-Transfusion Medicine, Anatomic and Clinical Pathology
- Cardiothoracic Radiology, Diagnostic Radiology
- Cardiovascular Disease, Internal Medicine
- Chemical Pathology, Anatomic and Clinical Pathology
- Child Abuse Pediatrics, Pediatrics
- Child and Adolescent Psychiatry, Psychiatry
- Child Neurology, Neurology
- Clinical Cardiac Electrophysiology, Internal Medicine
- Clinical Neurophysiology, Neurology
- Colon and Rectal Surgery
- Congenital Cardiac Surgery, Thoracic Surgery
- Craniofacial Surgery, Plastic Surgery
- Critical Care Medicine, Anesthesiology
- Critical Care Medicine, Internal Medicine
- Cytopathology, Anatomic and Clinical Pathology
- Dermatology
- Dermatopathology, Dermatology
- Developmental and Behavioral Pediatrics, Pediatrics
- Diagnostic Radiology
- Emergency Medicine
- Endocrinology, Diabetes, and Metabolism, Internal Medicine
- Endovascular Surgical Neuroradiology, Neurological Surgery

- Endovascular Surgical Neuroradiology, Neurology
- Endovascular Surgical Neuroradiology, Diagnostic Radiology
- Family Medicine/Family Practice
- Female Pelvic Medicine and Reconstructive Surgery, Obstetrics and Gynecology
- Foot and Ankle Orthopedics, Orthopedic Surgery
- Forensic Pathology, Anatomic and Clinical Pathology
- Forensic Psychiatry, Psychiatry
- Gastroenterology, Internal Medicine
- General Surgery
- Geriatric Medicine, Family Medicine/Family Practice
- Geriatric Medicine, Internal Medicine
- Geriatric Psychiatry, Psychiatry
- Hand Surgery, Orthopedic Surgery
- Hand Surgery, Plastic Surgery
- Hand Surgery, General Surgery
- Hematology, Internal Medicine
- Hematology, Anatomic and Clinical Pathology
- Hematology and Oncology, Internal Medicine
- Hospice and Palliative Medicine
- Infectious Disease
- Integrated Plastic Surgery
- Integrated Thoracic Surgery
- Integrated Vascular Surgery
- Internal Medicine
- Internal Medicine-Emergency Medicine
- Internal Medicine-Pediatrics
- Interventional Cardiology, Internal Medicine
- Medical Genetics
- Medical Microbiology, Anatomic and Clinical Pathology

- Medical Toxicology, Emergency Medicine
- Micrographic Surgery and Dermatologic Oncology, Dermatology
- Molecular Genetic Pathology, Medical Genetics
- Musculoskeletal Oncology, Orthopedic Surgery
- Musculoskeletal Radiology, Diagnostic Radiology
- Neonatal-Perinatal Medicine, Pediatrics
- Nephrology, Internal Medicine
- Neurological Surgery
- Neurology
- Neuromuscular Medicine, Neurology
- Neuromuscular Medicine, Physical Medicine and Rehabilitation
- Neuromuscular Medicine and Osteopathic Manipulative Medicine/Osteopathic Neuromusculoskeletal Medicine
- Neuropathology, Anatomic and Clinical Pathology
- Neuroradiology, Diagnostic Radiology
- Nuclear Medicine
- Nuclear Radiology, Diagnostic Radiology
- Obstetric Anesthesiology, Anesthesiology
- Obstetrics and Gynecology
- Oncology, Internal Medicine
- Ophthalmic Plastic and Reconstructive Surgery, Ophthalmology
- Ophthalmology
- Orthopedic Sports Medicine, Orthopedic Surgery
- Orthopedic Surgery
- Orthopedic Surgery of the Spine, Orthopedic Surgery
- Orthopedic Trauma, Orthopedic Surgery
- Otolaryngology
- Otology-Neurotology, Otolaryngology

- Pain Medicine, Anesthesiology
- Pain Medicine, Neurology
- Pain Medicine, Physical Medicine and Rehabilitation
- Pediatric Anesthesiology, Anesthesiology
- Pediatric Cardiology, Pediatrics
- Pediatric Critical Care Medicine, Pediatrics
- Pediatric Emergency Medicine, Emergency Medicine
- Pediatric Emergency Medicine, Pediatrics
- Pediatric Endocrinology, Pediatrics
- Pediatric Gastroenterology, Pediatrics
- Pediatric Hematology-Oncology, Pediatrics
- Pediatric Infectious Disease, Pediatrics
- Pediatric Nephrology, Pediatrics
- Pediatric Orthopedics, Orthopedic Surgery
- Pediatric Otolaryngology, Otolaryngology
- Pediatric Pathology, Anatomic and Clinical Pathology
- Pediatric Pulmonology, Pediatrics
- Pediatric Radiology, Diagnostic Radiology
- Pediatric Rheumatology, Pediatrics
- Pediatric Sports Medicine, Pediatrics
- Pediatric Surgery, General Surgery
- Pediatric Transplant Hepatology, Pediatrics
- Pediatric Urology, Urology
- Pediatrics
- Physical Medicine and Rehabilitation
- Plastic Surgery
- Preventive Medicine
- Psychiatry
- Pulmonary Disease, Internal Medicine

- Pulmonary Disease and Critical Care Medicine, Internal Medicine
- Radiation Oncology
- Reproductive Endocrinology and Infertility
- Rheumatology, Internal Medicine
- Sleep Medicine
- Spinal Cord Injury Medicine, Physical Medicine and Rehabilitation
- Sports Medicine, Emergency Medicine
- Sports Medicine, Family Medicine/Family Practice
- Sports Medicine, Internal Medicine
- Sports Medicine, Physical Medicine and Rehabilitation
- Surgical Critical Care, General Surgery
- Thoracic Surgery
- Transplant Hepatology, Internal Medicine
- Urology
- Vascular and Interventional Radiology, Diagnostic Radiology
- Vascular Surgery, General Surgery

I know most of you just skimmed through the last few pages, and that is fine. The point of including that list in the book was not to get you to read every word. It was to demonstrate just how many options there are out there for you. It is not a bad idea for you at some point to go through that list line by line and cross out each specialty you are no longer considering. That way you can be sure you at least considered everything available to you. One of my regrets about medical school was not looking more closely at Anesthesiology as a specialty. Although I doubt I would have chosen it over Emergency Medicine in the end, it probably should have been my second choice and I never realized that until late in my residency.

The list above is not even complete. There are many other subspecialties with recognized board certifications. In addition to those specialties and subspecialties listed above, just in my own specialty of Emergency Medicine there are official recognized board certifications in Critical Care Medicine, Emergency Medical Services, Hospice and Palliative Medicine,

Neurocritical Care, Pain Medicine, Sports Medicine, and Undersea and Hyperbaric Medicine. Emergency Medicine also offers fellowships in Wilderness Medicine, Ultrasound, and Administration, for which there are no official board certifications.

Feeling overwhelmed? I do not blame you. I had no idea this many specialties even existed when I was in medical school. Frankly, it is amazing that as many of us find our way into the right specialty as we do given how early in the process this decision must be made.

Here are a few tips that should help you to decide.

First, consider what you find interesting to learn about during the first two years of medical school. For instance, if you hated your neuroscience block, you are probably not going to enjoy neurology or neurosurgery.

Second, try to get exposure to the various specialties during the first couple of years of medical school. Just like you shadowed physicians as an undergraduate, you can similarly follow doctors around in clinic during medical school, you just need to be proactive and ask. Even the first month of medical school is not too early. This is especially important for those who think they may be interested in a specialty that is typically only offered as an elective at their school.

Third, try to find a good "fit." For example, I would attend many of the "Lunch and Learn" sessions put on by the various specialty interest groups at the school. Sure, the free pizza helped, but I was genuinely interested in learning more about specialties and specialists. I entered medical school thinking I was going into Family Medicine, but after attending a Lunch and Learn featuring an emergency physician during my second year, I realized I was more like that physician than any other doctor I had ever met. While there are many in every specialty who do not fit the stereotype of their specialty, there is a reason these stereotypes exist. Many emergency physicians actually are outdoorsy adrenaline junkies who love to travel. Many orthopedic surgeons actually are in the "500 Club." I better explain this one, since the USMLE Step 1 no longer reports board scores. Many orthopedic surgery residents would joke about being in the "500 Club," which meant their Step 1 score plus their maximum bench press in pounds was > 500. Many pathologists prefer not to interact with patients directly. Many surgeons are confident, action-oriented, workaholics who are not afraid to make a decision. This reminds me of the old duck hunting joke.

Five doctors went duck hunting one day. Included in the group was a family physician, a pediatrician, a psychiatrist, a surgeon, and a pathologist. A bird flew overhead and the first to react was the family physician, who raised his shotgun, but then hesitated.

"I'm not quite sure it's a duck," he said, "I think that I will have to get a second opinion." And of course by that time, the bird was long gone.

Another bird appeared in the sky soon thereafter. This time, the pediatrician drew a bead on it. He too, however, was unsure if it was really a duck in his sights and besides, it might have babies. "I'll have to do some more investigations," he muttered, as the creature made good its escape.

Next to spy a bird flying was the sharp-eyed psychiatrist. Shotgun shouldered, she was more certain of her intended prey's identity. "Now, I know it's a duck, but does it know it's a duck?" The fortunate bird disappeared while the lady wrestled with this dilemma.

Finally, a fourth fowl sped past and this time the surgeon's weapon pointed skywards and he fired without hesitation. BOOM! The surgeon lowered his smoking gun and turned nonchalantly to the pathologist beside him: "Go see if that was a duck, will you?"

Despite these stereotypes, you should not be afraid to buck a stereotype if a field interests you. There are plenty of people who hate rock climbing in Emergency Medicine and plenty of impressively social radiologists. Do not choose your specialty based on what other people think of the specialty, especially in the ivory towers of medicine—those tertiary referral centers where most of us trained. It is common to hear physicians in these centers, particularly resident physicians, denigrate their peers of other specialties. For example, an internal medicine intern might describe emergency physicians as "glorified triage nurses" based on experience acquired during a one-month rotation in an ivory tower emergency department (ED) during medical school. The intern might be surprised to learn that a community emergency physician typically discharges 85% of patients seen, serves as the chief of the medical staff, and rarely calls another specialist to the ED in person.

Fourth, consider the downsides of the specialty. Every specialty has a few downsides. If you do not know what they are, you have not spent enough time to rule it in or out. Pediatricians will tell you the worst part of their job is dealing with neurotic parents, for instance. Make sure that the downsides of your specialty do not bother you very much, or at least much less than they bother the typical doctor. For example, if you absolutely detest being on call, a career in General Surgery or Obstetrics is probably not a good idea. If it bothers you a great deal to take care of a homeless person with a serious addiction at 3 a.m., Emergency Medicine is likely not for you. If you do not actually enjoy doing procedures, Anesthesiology would be a poor choice.

Fifth, consider the bread and butter of the specialty. Most doctors spend the majority of their time taking care of just a handful of problems. For a general surgeon, this might include appendicitis, gallbladder disease, and hernias. An emergency physician easily spends 90% of clinical time taking care of patients with complaints of abdominal pain, chest pain, dyspnea, altered mental status, suicidal ideation, and vaginal bleeding. A general internist will be managing diabetes, hypertension, or hypercholesterolemia during most visits. If you do not like treating eczema and ruling out melanoma, you probably should not go into dermatology. Do you hate well-child checks and detest talking to parents about the benefits of immunizations? Pediatrics is not for you. Make sure you recognize and enjoy the bread and butter of your chosen specialty.

Now, with those preliminary remarks out of the way, let us remember that this is a financial book. I would be remiss not to discuss the financial ramifications of your specialty choice. I was surprised to do a poll of physicians a few years ago and learn that more than ¼ of doctors chose a specialty without any idea what the income or lifestyle of physicians in that specialty was like.[18] While I absolutely agree that this decision is not primarily a financial decision, that strikes me as piss-poor career planning for which there is no excuse whatsoever. So let us start with a simple chart (found on the next page) showing the average reported income for the various specialties. This list comes from the widely publicized 2020 Medscape Physician Compensation Report, a survey of over 17,000 physicians of various specialties.[19] The data is not perfect, but it will give you a general idea of the earning potential of the various specialties relative to one another.

Now you cannot say you were not warned. Do not be surprised that if you go into Preventive Medicine that you cannot drive as nice of a car, live in as fancy of a house, go on as nice of vacations, and retire as early as your friend who went into Plastic Surgery. That said, I think there are a few things you should recognize about physician pay.

First, recognize that these numbers are not static. From time to time, specialties move up and down this list. While Orthopedics has always been

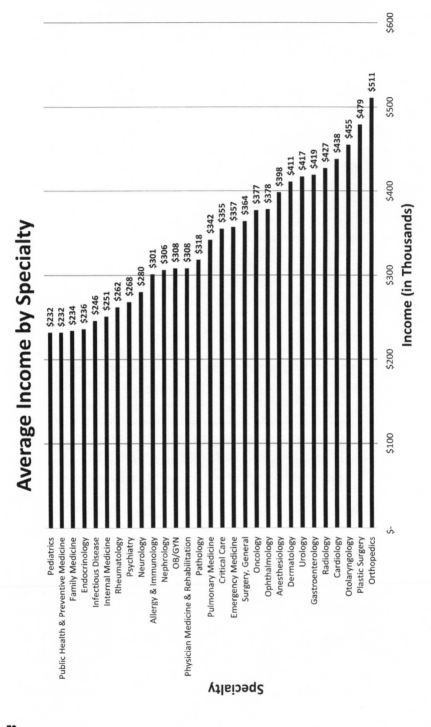

Average Income by Specialty

Specialty

Income (in Thousands)

Specialty	Income
Pediatrics	$232
Public Health & Preventive Medicine	$232
Family Medicine	$234
Endocrinology	$236
Infectious Disease	$246
Internal Medicine	$251
Rheumatology	$262
Psychiatry	$268
Neurology	$280
Allergy & Immunology	$301
Nephrology	$306
OB/GYN	$308
Physician Medicine & Rehabilitation	$308
Pathology	$318
Pulmonary Medicine	$342
Critical Care	$355
Emergency Medicine	$357
Surgery, General	$364
Oncology	$377
Ophthalmology	$378
Anesthesiology	$398
Dermatology	$411
Urology	$417
Gastroenterology	$419
Radiology	$427
Cardiology	$438
Otolaryngology	$455
Plastic Surgery	$479
Orthopedics	$511

in the top quartile and Pediatrics has always been in the bottom quartile, the list is not the same year to year.

Second, you should be aware that these are just averages. The actual range around these averages is very wide, far wider than you probably imagine in medical school. In fact, the intra-specialty pay differences are generally wider than the inter-specialty pay differences. I know of pediatricians making more than half a million dollars a year and I know of orthopedic surgeons making less than $150,000 per year. An emergency medicine salary survey from 2015 noted that the 10th percentile for employee emergency physicians was just $210,000 and the 90th percentile for partner emergency physicians was $510,000.[20] Statistics from other specialties show a similarly wide range.

Third, if you cannot live on a quarter-million dollars per year, you have a spending problem, not an earning problem. While not every physician job pays that much, it is not that hard to find a job as a physician of any specialty that will pay you that much money, although it may not be located in your desired city.

All of that said, your financial life will be much easier if you are in a specialty that makes more money. I am not going to lie to you and tell you it will be easy to pay off $550,000 in student loans as a family physician. It will not be. If you have a massive student loan burden, and are not willing to pursue a forgiveness program such as Public Service Loan Forgiveness, you may wish to cross out the lowest paying third of specialties on that list. In general, I feel medical students actually place too little weight on income potential and lifestyle when choosing a specialty. I assure you that you will care much more about those two factors 10 years out of residency than you will as an MS3. At least include them in your decision in some small way.

Hourly pay can be surprisingly variable. For example, a psychiatrist may earn $268,000 per year working 1,920 hours in that year. A surgeon may earn $364,000, but work 2,880 hours per year. At first glance, you might think the surgeon is more highly paid, but in reality the psychiatrist has a higher hourly wage ($140/hour versus $126/hour).

In addition, consider the training period. Some residencies are harder than others and post-graduate training periods can vary from three to seven years. A general surgeon, an emergency physician, and an intensivist all make similar amounts of money, but the surgeon trained for five years, the emergency doc for three, and the intensivist completed both a three-year residency and a three-year fellowship, for six years total. If one were to do a study of hourly pay somehow adjusted for the length of training, the list of specialties would likely be in a very different order. Every year of extra training is a year of lost attending income.

Some specialties are also more amenable to becoming a practice owner. A psychiatrist may need little more capital than a single room and two chairs and inexpensive malpractice insurance. An Oral and Maxillofacial Surgery (OMFS) clinic is going to require hundreds of thousands of dollars in capital and substantially higher malpractice premiums. While the general trend is toward more and more employees and fewer and fewer and fewer owners, the speed of that trend varies by specialty.

Some specialties lend themselves better to part-time work or side gigs than others. If you have a lot of interests outside of medicine like I did, you may want to give these specialties higher consideration. Specialties that lend themselves well to part-time work (usually the ones that do shift work such as Emergency Medicine, Anesthesiology, Radiology, and similar) can offer additional income opportunities or burn-out reducing flexibility. General or orthopedic surgery is much more difficult to do part-time, and it can be particularly hard to "escape from" a primary care practice where the patients all want to be seen by you. Dual-physician couples should consider how well their specialties will mesh together. Two neurosurgeons will likely have plenty of money, but may not be able to spend as much time together as they would like. Some specialties are also harder to practice in smaller towns where the cost of living is lower. Pediatric subspecialists or pathologists are not going to be able to work in the small towns they may have grown up in.

Still, the most important financial consideration of specialty choice is not the income potential. The most important factor is career longevity. You will be much better off financially practicing Endocrinology for 35 years than burning out of Radiology in 10. Not only will you have more total earnings, but you will pay a lower percentage of your earned income in taxes, have a larger Social Security benefit, and have more time for compound interest to work on your savings before you need to tap into that nest egg. So choose a specialty that you will love to practice for a long time, but for heaven's sake if you love Plastic Surgery and Infectious Disease equally, become a plastic surgeon.

MAIN IDEAS

- There are more specialties to choose from than most medical students realize.

- The most important financial aspect of specialty choice is career longevity.

- Know what the expected lifestyle and income is for each specialty.

- Even within a specialty, physicians have dramatically different incomes.

- Give at least some consideration to the financial ramifications of specialty choice. You will care far more about them later than you do now.

ADDITIONAL RESOURCES

- **Blog Post:** Picking a Specialty
  www.whitecoatinvestor.com/picking-a-specialty-friday-qa-series/

- **Blog Post:** Intra-Specialty Salary Differences
  www.whitecoatinvestor.com/intra-specialty-salary-differences-on-merritt-hawkins/

- **Podcast:** #158 Which Physician Specialty Is Best for Retiring Early?
  www.whitecoatinvestor.com/which-physician-specialty-is-best-for-retiring-early-podcast-158/

CHAPTER NINE

HOW TO CHOOSE A SPECIALTY (DENTISTS)

It might seem presumptuous of me, as a physician, to include a chapter in this book about how to choose a specialty as a dentist. However, this process is sufficiently unique that the previous chapter cannot simply be applied to the situation facing a graduating dental student. The decision to specialize, and if so which specialty to practice, will have a dramatic effect on the financial life of a dentist. Understanding the financial implications is critical to making the decision correctly in order to maximize career longevity, reduce burnout, boost earning potential, and minimize the direct and opportunity costs associated with the decision.

The first issue to address is whether you should specialize or not. Very few physicians do the minimum required one-year internship and then start practicing. Of those who do, the majority are in the military and eventually return to complete a full residency. This is not the case with dentists. The majority of dentists still complete no residency training at all. One can complete a professionally and financially successful career as a general dentist without spending a single day as a resident. These doctors are not necessarily "Medicaid or corporate dentists" either. Many are highly-profitable sole practitioners or even own multiple practices.

Two concerns should guide the decision to pursue specialty training. The first is what you want to do with the rest of your life. Just like with physicians choosing a specialty, this is a career we are talking about! You are likely to pour more of the best hours of your life into this profession than anything else that you will ever do. Ideally, your choice will be something that you love. The ideal career is one that you would do for free—that you will wake up each morning excited to do more than anything else. As the old saying goes, "Choose a career you love and you will never work a day in your life." However, let us be honest. Almost nobody will practice medicine, dentistry, or any of their specialties 40+ hours a week without any financial remuneration at all. It is called "work" because they have to pay you to do it. A while back, I surveyed a group of over 600 physicians and dentists, the vast majority of which were not financially independent, asking how much they would work if they had $10 million in the bank.[21] You may find the answers surprising.

How Much Would Doctors Work If They Did Not Need the Money?	
Hours per Week	% of Doctors
0	30.0%
1-10	3.7%
11-20	47.7%
21-30	14.0%
31-40	3.3%
41-50	0.5%
>50	0.8%

You might think that most doctors in that situation would not work at all. However, fewer than ⅓ of doctors would quit work completely despite having plenty of money. At the same time, very few would work anywhere near full-time, with less than one in 20 being willing to work more than 30 hours a week. A sizable majority would still work part-time, between 11 and 30 hours a week.

I cite this poll to demonstrate an important principle. That principle is that you will be working at least partly for the money. You need to come to peace with that and recognize that people are complex and are motivated by multiple factors. In our society, financial remuneration is a major way in which appreciation is shown. At the same time, I think it is just as important to recognize that people who go into professions like dentistry are not completely motivated by financial gain. In fact, I suspect they are less motivated than the vast majority by financial gain. What percentage of custodians or real estate agents do you suspect would still want to work 11–30 hours a week if they did not need the money?

So you obviously have to find a balance. Consider what you like doing with your day. The day to day work of an orthodontist, oral surgeon, pediatric dentist, or periodontist is significantly different from that of a general dentist. What do you like to study? Do you like doing the challenging cases that other doctors do not want to touch, or do you prefer knowing that you can refer out anything you do not want to do? Do you want to be dependent on general dentists for your patient flow, or do you prefer to go directly to the public?

The second concern that should guide the decision of whether to specialize or not should be the financial ramifications. Jonathan Clements, author and financial columnist, famously advises young people to place a great deal of emphasis on financial ramifications with their career choice:

> "When I talk to college students, I don't tell them to follow their dreams. Instead, I tell them to focus on making and saving money. I even suggest that they might deliberately opt for a less interesting but higher paying job, so they can sock away serious sums of money. All this might sound deadly dull and horribly reactionary. Aren't those in their 20s meant to pursue their passions, before they become burdened by the demands of raising a family and making the monthly mortgage payment? Underpinning this is an implicit—but rarely examined—assumption: that pursuing our passions is somehow more important in our 20s than in our 50s. I think this is nonsense. In fact, I think just the opposite is true."[22]

Choosing to specialize has serious financial ramifications, and since this is a financial book, we should probably spend some time discussing them. The main financial consideration boils down to a simplistic formula— how much more will you earn per year as a specialist than you would as a generalist and, if so, does that overcome the costs, including opportunity cost, of becoming a specialist?

So let us address the first part of that. Will you earn more as a specialist, and if so, how much more? The ADA Health Policy Institute publishes the reported incomes of generalist and specialist dentists each year. At the time of writing of this chapter, the most up to date data comes from the year 2018. Every dental student should be familiar with this data, so I will recreate the main table from the survey here:[23]

Type of Dentist	Average	1st Quartile	Median	3rd Quartile
General Practitioners				
All Owners	$201,860	$120,000	$175,000	$250,000
Solo	$187,810	$110,000	$158,000	$240,000
Nonsolo	$235,720	$142,500	$200,000	$300,000
Employed	$160,110	$95,000	$150,000	$191,000
All General Practitioners	**$190,440**	**$110,000**	**$160,000**	**$250,000**
Specialists				
All Owners	$356,670	$200,000	$300,000	$475,000
Solo	$340,250	$180,000	$300,000	$450,000
Nonsolo	$378,230	$216,000	$350,000	$500,000
Employed	$257,280	$165,000	$220,000	$344,000
All Specialists	**$330,180**	**$180,000**	**$280,000**	**$406,000**
All Dentists				
All Owners	$233,840	$120,000	$200,000	$300,000
Solo	$214,190	$120,000	$175,000	$275,000
Nonsolo	$275,240	$150,000	$250,000	$360,000
Employed	$184,790	$108,000	$160,000	$230,000
All Dentists	**$220,950**	**$120,000**	**$180,000**	**$280,000**

As you can see, the median generalist earned $160,000 per year and the median specialist earned $280,000 per year. There are two worthwhile lessons to take from that information. First, specialists do get paid more than generalists, which opens up the possibility that specializing may pay off financially. Second, the median dentist, whether a generalist or a specialist, does not make all that much money compared to the highest-earning dentists. Everybody knows of an orthodontist or an oromaxillofacial surgeon (OMFS) with a seven-figure income. It is important to realize upfront that only a minority of dental specialists have such lucrative practices. That does not mean you cannot become one of those folks, but you need to understand it is not even close to guaranteed. Another lesson that can be learned from that data is that those willing to take on the burdens and risks of practice ownership earn more than those who do not, at least on average. We will address this in a later chapter.

The incomes of the various dental specialists are highly variable. The data from the ADA survey is further broken down by specialty as follows.

Type of Dentist	Average	1st Quartile	Median	3rd Quartile
Oral Maxillofacial Surgeons	$420,020	$274,820	$375,000	$500,000
Endodontists	$342,950	$200,000	$318,000	$425,000
Orthodontists	$353,790	$200,000	$300,000	$450,000
Pediatric Dentists	$287,040	$150,000	$220,000	$400,000
Periodontists	$268,830	$150,000	$250,000	$350,000
Prosthodontists	$233,550	$130,000	$195,000	$280,000

Again, the data demonstrates some important points. First, the obvious point that OMFS and orthodontic specialists earn far more than pediatric and prosthodontic specialists. Second, there is quite a wide range of income within any given specialty. Just like in medicine, the intra-specialty income range is much wider than the inter-specialty income range. Finally, note that many specialists actually earn less than many generalists! Specialization is not a guaranteed path to a higher income! When running the numbers for your own personal situation, you must consider what you will earn as a specialist versus what you will earn as a generalist, rather than simply what the median doctor will get.

Unfortunately, when you run your numbers, you cannot simply use gross income to help you make the specialization decision. Since high-income professionals often face substantial tax burdens, you must first adjust the numbers for taxes. While tax burden is highly variable by state, family situation, employment situation, and other factors, you can generally assume that an orthodontist earning $300,000 per year will pay a higher percentage of her income in taxes than a generalist earning $160,000 per year. It might be reasonable to project that the generalist will pay 18% in taxes and the orthodontist 25%. So the after-tax incomes that you should actually be comparing would be $131,200 to $225,000, a difference of only $93,800 rather than $140,000.

Now, let us consider the costs of specialization. The first of these is the actual cost of doing a residency. Many physicians are flabbergasted to learn that many dental residencies not only do not pay a salary, but actually charge tuition! This is highly variable, but the most remunerative specialties are the most likely to charge higher tuition. For example, almost all orthodontic residencies charge tuition, but it varies from as little as $2,000 per year to as much as $116,000 per year for the three-year program. Since residency is three years long, the loan burden from residency can be just as large as the loan burden from dental school itself, which is already higher than that faced by the average physician.

The second cost of specialization is the interest cost. Most dentists use student loans to pay for dental school. The interest from those loans will continue to grow during residency training. Simple interest at 7% on $400,000 in student loans is $28,000 per year, or $92,000 over the course of a three-year residency. If that debt is paid off over the next 10 years, the total additional interest that will be paid as a result of doing the residency would be about $83,000.

The third cost of specializing is the opportunity cost of not practicing as a generalist for the three years you will be in residency. If the average generalist makes $131,200 after-tax, that adds up to about $394,000.

If we assume a residency tuition of $60,000 per year ($180,000 total), $92,000 in additional interest costs, and $394,000 in opportunity cost, we see that the cost of specializing is approximately $666,000. With a median earning differential of $93,800 after-tax, we see that the breakeven point is approximately seven years out of residency or 10 years out of dental school. Thus, in this scenario with these assumptions, it will eventually pay off to become an orthodontist. However, it does not take much monkeying around with the assumptions to push that break-even point out another decade or two, especially in the less lucrative specialties. In a worst-case scenario, it may not pay off at all! Although, most of the time specializing, assuming you love the specialty, is probably going to pay off eventually.

Unfortunately, there is another issue involved in choosing to specialize. You may not be able to do it even if you want to. Some specialties are more competitive than others in medicine, but all specialties are competitive in dentistry. Only 21% of dentists are specialists, and anecdotally, the vast majority of specialists were in the top quartile of their graduating classes and had excellent board scores. Even if the school has a pass/fail grading system, there are often specialty-specific tests you must take, such as the Comprehensive Basic Science Exam (CBSE) for OMFS. The match rates are often lower than even the most competitive specialties in medicine—and remember that many people who would like to do a specialty do not even bother applying after sizing up their own competitiveness. In 2020, specialty match rates were as follows:[24]

Dental Specialist Match Rates	
Specialty	Match Rate
Pediatric Dentistry	61%
Orthodontics	61%
Dental Anesthesia	54%
Oral Maxillofacial Surgeons	53%
Prosthodontics	45%
Periodontics	43%

Endodontics statistics are harder to come by, as they do not go through the regular dental match, but the specialty is also generally considered to be highly competitive.

Once you have decided to specialize, carefully consider the decision just as a physician would. Try to get as much exposure to those specialists and the procedures they do as you can and try to determine what you most enjoy. As I told the physicians, if you enjoy two specialties equally and think you can match into either, choose the one that makes more financial sense!

As long as we are talking about residency training, we should discuss the two types of generalist residencies, the General Practice Residency (GPR) and the Advanced Education in General Dentistry (AEGD) programs. These programs can also be competitive to match into, with 2020 match rates of

64% and 44% respectively.[25] Both programs are generally one year long, but can extend to two years.

The GPR is hospital-based and allows a dentist to gain hospital privileges. The dentist rotates on the medical Internal Medicine, Surgery, and Anesthesia services as well as various dental specialties. The emphasis is on medical management. Think of it as learning how to do dentistry on medically complex patients.

The AEGD is clinic-based—a bit more like an additional year of dental school but with more autonomy. Both programs are thought to provide experience equal to several years of clinical practice and are growing in popularity. Also, both tend to pay stipends, rather than charge tuition like many of the specialty training programs. Some states, such as Delaware and New York, require a residency to be completed, but most still do not. Thus, there is significant regional variation in whether dentists do residencies or not. In the Northeast, they are quite common. On the West coast, not so much. The value of these residencies will continue to be controversial. Some dentists who reviewed this book clearly viewed them as a waste of a year. Like anything in life, those who did them view them more positively than those who did not.

Residency training may also make you a more competitive candidate for a job, resulting in a higher salary. I was unable to find any good data demonstrating a definite financial benefit, but since it is usually only one year and you may be paid a salary of $40,000–$60,000 as you do it, the cost of doing the training is so minor that it should not be a primarily financial decision. If you want or need the training, get it. If you do not, you should not feel badly about going straight into practice.

At the end of the day, dental specialization is generally a good idea for your finances. If you want to practice a specialty, can match into a position, and practice for most or all of a career, it should pay off. That said, run the numbers for yourself and do your best to match into a program that pays a stipend, or at least charges a low rate of tuition.

MAIN IDEAS

- Many dental residencies not only do not pay you, but charge you tuition.

- Specializing is much less common for dentists than physicians.

- Specialization generally increases income.

- The decision to specialize as a dentist has financial ramifications, but should primarily be made based on non-financial factors.

ADDITIONAL RESOURCES

- **Blog Post:** Debt Dilemmas for Dental Specialists *www.whitecoatinvestor.com/debt-dilemmas-for-dental-specialists/*

CHAPTER TEN

AVOIDING FINANCIAL CATASTROPHES

Financial catastrophes are events that are so large that they set you back for years or even decades in your progression toward your financial goals. There are many financial catastrophes. Some you can insure against and some you cannot.

Financial Catastrophes You Can Insure Against

Professional liability

Personal liability

Loss of valuable personal property

Disability

Death of a breadwinner with dependents

Serious illness or injury

Financial Catastrophes You Cannot Insure Against

Divorce

Gambling or drug addiction

Loss of licensure or hospital privileges

Career change from Medicine or Dentistry

Failure to match

Failure to pass the bar exam

Too many Americans, including doctors, buy insurance to protect against financial loss that would not actually be a financial catastrophe (consider how many people buy Applecare® for their iPhone). Meanwhile, they do not bother purchasing term life or disability insurance and carry only the state-required minimum liability insurance. So make sure you protect against those financial catastrophes that can be insured against by purchasing personal (umbrella) and professional (malpractice) liability policies, homeowner's or renter's insurance, disability insurance, term life insurance if you have dependents, and health insurance. It is reasonable to put some of those insurance policies (liability, disability) off until your intern year rather than purchase them with borrowed money, but a medical or dental student could certainly justify buying an inexpensive term life policy during school, and everyone needs health insurance.

In this chapter, I am going to focus on the uninsurable financial catastrophes, particularly career change and the failure to match. The other catastrophes deserve at least a paragraph apiece though.

Divorce, while less common among doctors than the general population, is one of the biggest catastrophes out there—and the later in life it happens, the bigger deal it becomes, at least financially-speaking. A typical physician divorce cuts your net worth and your future income, at least for a few years, in half. Thus a doctor's best asset protection move might be date night! Consider a pre-nuptial agreement, especially if marrying after developing substantial income or acquiring significant wealth, and certainly if there are children from a previous marriage. You might even consider a post-nuptial agreement if both spouses are willing. Divorce law is state-specific. Some states are friendlier to men, and others to women. "Standard" alimony calculations can be surprisingly different in some states versus others. As a general rule, a medical student or resident who gets divorced will not owe as much in alimony as an attending physician who gets divorced. Many divorcees express regret at not getting better advice prior to initiating proceedings. They also universally advise that both spouses always be involved in managing the money, no matter how busy one might be as a student or resident. They also recommend pre-marital counseling.

One early reviewer of this book noted that female doctors have a 50% higher divorce rate than male doctors. She said being a doctor is stressful by itself, but even worse when you also become a single mother paying alimony, especially if you are not being paid as well as your male peers.

She recommends that women doctors learn to advocate for themselves, find mentors, and take leadership classes.

Now I joked about date night above, but its importance cannot be overstated. While I am serious about the financial benefits, those pale in comparison to the mental, social, and emotional benefits you will enjoy from an optimized relationship. Your relationship is likely to be the greatest contributor to your lifelong happiness. Prioritize and protect it.

Gambling or drug addiction in you or your partner is another great way to lose your income or wealth. Get help if you have this issue and always stay involved enough in the family finances that any issue with your spouse cannot be hidden for long. This can be perhaps the most serious form of financial infidelity.

Many doctors do not realize that malpractice insurance only covers one of your many professional liabilities. Your malpractice policy will not pay a thing in the event of one of these other professional risks:

Medicare or Medicaid fraud

Accusations of sexual harassment of staff members

Accusations of inappropriate patient relationships

Loss of licensure

Loss of hospital privileges

Inappropriate alteration of medical records

Criminal acts

Each of these can result in simultaneous lawsuits and loss of income, but you cannot insure against any of them. Be on your best behavior, and develop habits that will protect you in the event of false accusation. Physicians and dentists are placed in a trusted position in society; do not betray that trust. Aside from your reputation, you could lose millions of dollars.

However, this book is written for the medical or dental student, so I want to focus on student-specific financial catastrophes. In the last decade or two the price of your education has soared dramatically. Most students are going into significant debt for their education, often finishing their training owing $200,000, $300,000, $400,000, or more in student loans. I have even run into a few dental specialists who owe over a million dollars in student loans.

When racking up this sort of debt, anything that eliminates your ability to finish your training and practice in your chosen field, at least for a few years, becomes a financial catastrophe.

This is unfortunate, because it can be impossible to predict what you, as a 21-year-old undergraduate student taking the MCAT or DAT, will enjoy or what you are good at in a decade or two. While most medical and dental students will love their education and feel fulfilled to finally be learning something they will use for the rest of their careers (instead of organic chemistry), there is a significant minority who will find medicine or dentistry is not what they thought it would be. Or worse, they are struggling academically. Imagine being two or three years into your education, already $200,000–$300,000 in debt, and realizing that you hate it? It happens every year to a handful of students in every class. Or perhaps you do not hate it, but you are seriously struggling, failing classes repeatedly and dropping from one class to the next to the next as you repeat mandatory classes and rotations.

Sometimes a medical student can slip through the classes, passing them all but never excelling. He arrives at the end of school with poor grades and mediocre board scores. Then he discovers on match day that he has not matched into his chosen specialty...or any specialty. While a dentist can go directly into practice, that is not an option for a physician and each year the medical schools in this country produce hundreds of doctors who will never be able to practice.

Each of these scenarios involves great disappointment and psychological struggles. But when combined with the massive debt acquired by most students, it also becomes an almost insurmountable financial catastrophe. While a doctor can generally earn enough to pay off her student loans, there are very few other career fields that can out-earn a doctor's student loans! A few words of advice are appropriate for each scenario.

First, I will address students who realize they do not actually want to finish school or become a doctor anymore. Realize that this is a common thought that nearly every professional student will have at some point in their education or training. Be careful not to make a rash decision. Give great thought to what has changed since you enrolled as an excited first-year student. Do not drop out of school in reaction to poor performance in one class or rotation. Do not let anyone else push you out with inappropriate harassment. If you are struggling with a physical or mental health issue (depression, anxiety, substance abuse, and ADHD are all common among professional students), see a qualified professional and seek out supportive peers in person and online. No matter what the issue might be, involve your dean's office early. You will not be the first person at your school considering leaving and they have access to resources and ideas you may not have even considered.

If you are sure you do not want to practice medicine or dentistry as a career, consider the stage of your education that you are currently at. If you are only in the first or second year, your debt burden may not yet be particularly large. While it is unfortunate to owe $50,000–$100,000, there are still lots of career fields that a person smart and motivated enough to get into medical or dental school can use to pay off those student loans. However, if you are in your third or fourth year, you may be looking at leaving school with several hundred thousand dollars in debt and no realistic ability to pay it back.

A person in this scenario should be aware of all of their options. First, realize that having an MD, DO, DDS, or DMD behind your name has some value, even if you never do a day of residency training. These are difficult and respected degrees that can open many doors that would otherwise be closed to you. Research, industry, and even academia is looking for people with that degree to perform unique, non-clinical tasks. So consider finishing the degree for financial reasons, even if you are not enjoying it. Unlike when I was in medical school, there are now entire organizations, books, and conferences dedicated to non-clinical careers for doctors such as Dr. Sylvie Stacy's excellent book simply titled *50 Nonclinical Careers for Physicians*.[26]

Also, recognize that every year of additional post-graduate training comes with significant earning potential. A doctor who completes only their intern year can get a license and practice as a general practitioner or in an urgent care type situation. Just because you complete a residency does not mean you have to practice and just because you practice for a few years does not mean you have to do it the rest of your career. In fact, I suspect the most common pathway for someone who realizes late in medical school (or even in residency) that they do not really want to do medicine, is to complete medical school, complete residency, practice for a few years, pay off their student loans, and then change careers or open their own business. The new career may or may not be medically related, but if you can get that far, you have certainly eliminated any financial catastrophe you would have been facing to drop out as an MS3. There are entire organizations of doctors dedicated to assisting other doctors who want to transition to a peripherally related or even completely unrelated field. I assure you that you will not be alone on your pathway.

Next, let us address the student who is academically struggling. It seems that medical and dental school admissions offices are putting less and less weight on academic credentials such as science GPA and MCAT/DAT scores each year. Rather than looking for the most academically qualified, the goal now seems to be to find students who are academically adequate, but excelling in other "softer" skills and attributes like communication, compassion, service, career goals, and background. This shift may not necessarily be a bad thing (nor is it particularly new, since it was the way our admissions committee operated when I was on it as an MS4 in 2002), but it does come with consequences, including having a few students that will academically struggle. You may find yourself in this boat.

Involve your dean's office early. Medical schools generally do not want to "weed out" any of their students. Your failure to graduate is also viewed as their failure. Tutoring, support, and additional time to complete your studies is likely available, and often at no additional cost to you. Spending three years instead of the traditional two to complete the pre-clinical years and pass Step 1 of the boards may be all you need to pass your classes and the test. The bar to success will soon be a little lower now that the USMLE (the licensing exam series for doctors) Step 1 exam has been converted to a pass/fail test, in that prospective residency programs will never know you barely passed. Many students who struggle in the pre-clinical years will do just fine on their rotations and into residency. If you find yourself struggling on clinical rotations, the process is similar. If you are humble and motivated, the school will likely find a way to get you sufficiently educated, even if it takes a little more time.

Recognize that you will probably be excluded from the more competitive specialties. A dentist is probably not going to become an endodontist after graduating at the bottom of the class, and a low-achieving medical student is not going to get into dermatology or orthopedics either. That is okay, there are many rewarding and necessary fields in medicine that for whatever reason are not as popular. Remember the old joke,

"What do you call someone who graduates at the bottom of their medical school class?"

"Doctor."

Focus your specialty selection decision on the less competitive fields, apply and interview more broadly than the average student, and develop relationships with faculty members who can write you a fantastic letter of recommendation extolling your non-academic attributes!

One of the most significant financial catastrophes for a medical student often comes as a sudden surprise. On Monday morning of Match Week, they get a call from the dean's office informing them that they did not match. This gut-wrenching experience is common and becoming more so each year as the number of medical students increases at a faster rate than the number of residency slots available. You might be surprised to learn that it has not always been this way. Up until the 70s, there were actually more residency positions than there were graduating students. However, now there are only about 77 positions for every 100 applicants. That overall match rate, however, hides an important fact—where you go to school has a dramatic effect on your likelihood of matching. Consider statistics from the 2020 NRMP Match, i.e. the match for MD students.[27]

Medical Specialist Match Rates (MD Match)	
Type of Student	Match Rate
US MD School, First Try	94%
US MD School, 2nd or Later Try	46%
US DO School, 1st Try	91%
US DO School, 2nd or Later Try	43%
International MD School	61%

As you can see, while the overall match rate may be only 77%, almost 19 out of 20 of those who graduate from a US MD school are going to match on their first try. A fair number of those folks who did not match would have matched, had they applied to and interviewed at more programs or sought out a less competitive specialty.

The DO statistics are particularly interesting. The match rate of DOs in the MD match has climbed dramatically in the last few years. As recently as 2016, that rate was only 84% on the first try and 37% on a 2nd or later try. You should be aware that the DO match rate in the DO match is much higher, over 98%.[27] So many of those DOs who do not match into an MD program simply train in a DO program and do not face a financial catastrophe.

The real tragedy in these statistics, however, is seen among international graduates. These students often attend expensive Caribbean medical schools that may not even qualify for federal student loans with their lower interest rates and various protective features. It can be a real gamble to attend one of these "2nd Chance Medical Schools," rack up $400,000 or more in student loans, and then hope you are one of the three out of five that will actually match. When applying to these schools, pay special attention to the match rates and the specialties that their graduates match into. Some schools have a better track record than others, but none of them are even close to the worst US MD schools. If you are struggling to get into medical school, you are generally far better off attending a DO school than a Caribbean school.

So what do you do if you do not match? The obvious first answer is to apply again. Meet with the dean's office, your faculty advisor(s), and the program director at your institution in your desired specialty, if available. Figure out what happened. Maybe you did a poor job of applying and interviewing and simply needed to cast a broader net. Maybe you overestimated your competitiveness for that specialty and need to lower your sights. Maybe with some additional research or rotations you will be a more competitive applicant. Use this additional year wisely to make yourself more competitive and apply to every single program in your desired specialty the second year. Go to every interview you get. Perhaps also apply to a less competitive "back-up" specialty or "PGY1-only" positions, so at least you can obtain licensure. While students that did not match the first time are certainly less likely to match the second time, almost half of them do. Do what you can to be in that half!

Obviously, if this occurs to you as a dentist, the consequences are much less dramatic. You simply go into practice, usually as an associate. You can apply again the next year or in a few years if you so desire. But if you are a medical school graduate and still have not matched after two or three tries, it is time to find a new career. Hopefully, you can leverage the MD or DO degree in some way.

But what should you do about the student loans? You cannot simply declare bankruptcy, because student loans do not go away in bankruptcy. If all or most of your student loans are federal student loans, you have some great options to have affordable payments and even have the loans forgiven. The best option is usually Public Service Loan Forgiveness. If you make 120 on-time monthly payments on qualifying loans in a qualifying program while employed full-time by a government or non-profit employer, the remainder of the federal student loans will be forgiven tax-free. When combined with an Income-Driven Repayment (IDR) program such as Income-Based Repayment (IBR), Pay As You Earn (PAYE), or Revised Pay As You Earn (REPAYE), you can have affordable monthly payments and never have to pay back the vast majority of your loan burden. If I could not match out of medical school, this is the route I would take. I would only consider jobs that would qualify for PSLF. 10 years out of medical school, I would be out of debt. You will be out of debt before many of your practicing physician colleagues!

There are other forgiveness programs associated with the various IDR programs. However, these are not nearly as attractive. Although they do not require you to work full-time for a government or non-profit employer (in fact they do not require you to work at all), they require you to make payments for 20–25 years and more importantly, the forgiveness is fully taxable at ordinary income tax rates in the year you receive it. If you thought it was hard to pay off medical school loans on a non-physician salary, imagine having to pay the taxes on $800,000 you never received all in one year on a non-physician salary! So while the IDR programs certainly help you in the short run by minimizing the payments (or even eliminating them if your income is low enough or you are unemployed), in the long run they may not be the best option if you do not have the ability to deal with that tax bomb. If you thought owing money to the Department of Education was bad, wait until you owe it to the Internal Revenue Service.

For attorneys, not passing the bar exam causes a similar outcome to not matching as a physician. Bar passage rates vary by school (from 20% to more than 98%) and by state (from 44% to 79%). Failure to pass the bar seems to be happening more and more frequently. Some attribute it to the rise in for-profit or unaccredited law schools. Other factors may include certain policies admitting students with lower LSAT scores or perhaps deliberately lower bar exam passage rates. No matter what the cause, without passing the bar it can become very difficult to acquire a job that pays enough to cover your debts.

Obviously studying hard and taking the bar exam again and again should be your first approach. You might have a JD, but you cannot call yourself an attorney, much less practice law, until you pass the bar. There are legal jobs available to you, however. These are sometimes called "JD Advantage Careers," because those with a law school degree have an advantage in getting the job over other applicants. Estimates are that approximately 15% of law school graduates take one of these JD Advantage jobs. The jobs include contract administrator, mediator, arbitrator, regulatory or compliance analyst, legal writer or editor, law firm or law school administrator, and management consultant. Just like an MD or DO, a JD can be a useful degree, even if you do not ever practice your profession.

So if you leave school with a substantial loan burden due to lack of interest, lack of ability, or inability to match or pass the bar, you need to find a way to take care of those loans. If family cannot help, you do not expect an inheritance any time soon, and you do not expect to marry someone with substantial wealth or at least a much higher income, there are really only two good choices. The first is to find another career that pays well enough to eventually pay off your student loans, or at least make the IDR payments while saving up enough for that tax bomb in a couple of decades. The second is to take a job with an employer that will qualify you for PSLF. I wish there were better options, but that is today's reality. Personally, I think some of this responsibility should be placed on the medical school. Maybe they should refund half of your tuition if you do not match, but I have not seen any legislation that would mandate that and I doubt we will ever see them do it voluntarily. I hope you never need the information in this chapter, but if you do, know that you are hardly alone and that others have successfully trod this path before you. There is light at the end of the tunnel.

MAIN IDEAS

- Financial catastrophes affect far too many physicians.

- Insurance, preparation, hard work, and good decision making can reduce the likelihood of a financial catastrophe.

- If you discover you are no longer in love with your chosen profession, consider finishing your training and rapidly paying off your student loans before pursuing another.

- If you fail to match in your chosen specialty, apply again using extreme care.

- Consider a PSLF-qualifying job to eliminate a massive loan burden associated with a career change.

ADDITIONAL RESOURCES

- **Blog Post:** One House, One Spouse, One Job
  www.whitecoatinvestor.com/one-house-one-spouse-one-job/

- **Blog Post:** Insure Only Against Financial Catastrophe
  www.whitecoatinvestor.com/insuring-against-catastrophes

- **Blog Post:** Big Debt Without an Income – A Med School Disaster
  www.whitecoatinvestor.com/big-debt-without-an-income-a-med-school-disaster/

- **Blog Post:** Physician Burnout: Factors and Cures
  www.whitecoatinvestor.com/physician-burnout-factors-cures/

- **Book:** *50 Nonclinical Careers for Physicians*[26]

CHAPTER ELEVEN

PREVENTING AND COMBATING BURNOUT

It may seem odd to include a chapter about burning out in a book aimed at those who have not yet officially started the career. However, burnout has become such a prevalent problem in medicine that every student needs to be aware of its existence, its causes, and especially its prevention and treatment from the very beginning.

There are some folks out there who do not really believe in burnout, or at least think a great deal of it is simply the tendency of folks to find something to complain about. Medicine has been criticized over the years for "medicalizing" a lot of conditions that are not actually medical conditions, and that criticism has extended to burnout. Critics might call it "medicalizing stress." "We all have stress and it makes our lives unpleasant," they say, "but that does not make it some sort of medical condition." The International Classification of Disease, the official compendium of diseases, now calls burnout "a syndrome resulting from chronic workplace stress."[28]

Richard Friedman wrote in a column in *The New York Times* stating that such a broad definition can apply to just about everybody and tells the story of a friend who took a wellness survey for her job. She answered yes to one question, whether she ever felt irritable at work, and was given the result that she was at risk of burnout. He argues that when a disorder is reportedly so widespread, it trivializes it. "If almost everyone suffers from burnout, then no one does, and the concept loses all credibility," he argues.[29]

Perhaps most famously, Yahoo! CEO Marissa Mayer argued, "I don't really believe in burnout. A lot of people work really hard for decades and decades, like Winston Churchill and Einstein," she said. Avoiding burnout has nothing to do with making sure you eat three square meals a day or get eight hours of sleep a night. "Burnout is about resentment," she said. "It's about knowing what matters to you so much that if you don't get it you're resentful." She argues that people can work many hard hours and not get burned out, so long as they are not forced to miss things that matter to them more than work.[30]

Others argue that a job is not supposed to provide some sense of philosophical self-actualization; it is supposed to provide a paycheck to put a roof over your head, clothes on your back, and food on your table. They say it is called work because it is so unpleasant that you have to be paid to do it. They say, "Feeling burned out at work? There is a support group for that; it meets Friday night down at the bar."

While I agree that cheapening and broadening the definition of burnout can cause some unintended consequences, the phenomenon is certainly real and medicine is a perfect laboratory to produce it. Burnout has been described as a workplace issue, and high-income professionals like physicians, dentists, and attorneys do not just clock in and out at a "9-to-5er," enjoy a classic lunch break every day, or even get all of their weekends off. Their workplace readily bleeds over into the rest of their life, so the severity of this "workplace issue" in these professions should not be terribly surprising.

Burnout is a chronic process of cynicism, exhaustion, decreased work performance, and powerlessness, caused by a disconnect between job demands, job resources, and the worker's ability to recover. To make matters worse, it seems to be closely connected to depression and suicide.

Medscape surveyed physicians in 2020 about burnout and suicide. The statistics provided by the survey are alarming. More than ⅔rds of physicians reported that burnout had a moderate to severe impact on their life. In answer to a simple question, "Are you burned out?" 42% of doctors answered, "Yes." Burnout is more common in women than men in medicine. It is currently more common among Generation X (mid-career docs) than Millennials (early-career docs) or Boomers (late-career docs). While it varies by specialty, even the least burned out specialty (Preventive Medicine) reports 29% of its practitioners are burned out. Interestingly, in recent years Urology,

Neurology, and Nephrology seem to have taken over from Emergency Medicine and Critical Care at the top of the list.[31]

When asked to identify the causes of their burnout, physicians list the following frequent job-related complaints:

Too many bureaucratic tasks (charting, paperwork): 55%

Spending too much time at work: 33%

Lack of respect from administrators, employers, colleagues, and staff: 32%

Increasing computerization of practice (EHRs): 30%

Insufficient compensation: 29%

Lack of control, autonomy: 24%

Feeling like a cog in the wheel: 22%

Decreasing reimbursements: 19%

Lack of respect from patients: 17%

Government regulations: 16%

Burnout is not just depression either, as only about 16% of doctors reported feeling depressed in the survey. However, the conditions often co-exist, resulting in alarming rates of suicidal ideation (23%) among physicians taking the survey. Physician suicide rates are double those of the general population. Nearly every doctor knows a student from their school or resident from their hospital who has killed himself or herself. The combination of high rates of suicidal ideation with an extensive knowledge of physiology, pathology, and pharmacology, and a culture where reporting any sort of mental illness has real reputational, professional, and financial consequences is a lethal combination. Many physicians have difficulty recognizing they are depressed. Mental illness still has a lot of stigma in our society. Perhaps it feels better to be burned out (meaning you have been working very hard) as opposed to depressed (meaning there is "something wrong with you").

Perhaps the most concerning question from the Medscape survey asked doctors how they coped with burnout. Many of the top answers included unhealthy behaviors such as isolating oneself, binge eating junk food, drinking alcohol, smoking, and using drugs—although exercising and sleeping were also high on the list.

Now this is a financial book, so I am going to focus a bit more on the financial aspects of burnout than you might see elsewhere. In my opinion, there are four contributors to burnout, although it is difficult to determine which of these most impacts any given person or even the doctor population as a whole. These four are:

- The stresses of medicine and dentistry
- Toxic jobs
- Inadequate personal resilience
- Financial factors

Interestingly, better financial planning can be part of the solution to all four problems.

The first of these factors is perhaps the hardest to do anything about. Medicine and dentistry will always be difficult, stressful professions. They require long periods of initial and ongoing education and training, long hours, interactions with difficult patients, and being around the seriously ill and injured. None of these are likely to go away, nor are profession-related issues like electronic health records, pre-qualifications, and the maintenance demands of board certification and credentialing. The only real escape from this factor is to practice medicine less or leave the profession completely. However, many physicians feel trapped in the profession by their financial circumstances. Whether a large student loan burden or an inflated lifestyle, since most careers pay less than medicine or dentistry, significant financial resources and discipline are required just to cut back, much less leave entirely. Only about half of physicians in the Medscape survey were willing to give up any pay at all in order to have a better work-life balance. Nevertheless, developing financial literacy and discipline while applying both to your physician salary over a matter of years can certainly provide options to reduce the impact of this factor on personal burnout, up to and including leaving the career for another or for no career at all.

Burnout specialists frequently talk about how burnout is a systemic or even an employer-specific problem. Certainly, burnout is contagious among a large group of doctors. There is no doubt that a major contributor to burnout is what I call a toxic or abusive job. This includes jobs with too much volume for staffing levels, inadequate support staff, one-sided contracts, malignant personalities, and unrealistic expectations. While these jobs can be changed, changes generally require at least a credible threat of leaving for another job. If you keep your financial ducks in a row, you can afford the loss of income that a job change usually involves. This provides you the leverage to force change if possible, and follow through on the threat of leaving if change is not possible.

Many of those who study or have burnout prefer to downplay the impact of personal resilience on burnout. However, it is a weak argument to say that personal factors have no impact whatsoever on burnout. Not all of the doctors in a given specialty in a given organization are burned out, so personal resilience does play at least some role. Solutions to this factor include medical care, therapy, diet, exercise, yoga, and meditation. However, perhaps the best way to improve personal resilience is simply to work less. Any time I meet a burned-out doctor, the first thing I recommend is that they cut back to full-time! Almost nobody can avoid burnout while working 60 or 80 hours a week year after year after year. Cutting back to 40 or 50 hours a week provides the time to do the activities that increase personal resilience. When surveyed, very few doctors would leave medicine completely if they were given $10 million dollars. But nearly every one of them would work less.[32] Financial planning can improve personal resilience because it provides the resources and ability to cut back on call, drop shifts, work less, and focus on the patients and procedures you enjoy most.

Finally, many doctors have financial stress in their lives. They feel like hamsters running on a treadmill to make next month's student loan, mortgage, and car payments. A surprising percentage of doctors live hand-to-mouth, essentially spending every dollar they make every month. When your finances feel out of control, it forces you to focus more on your financial needs than the needs of the patient in front of you. I am convinced that financially secure doctors are better partners, parents, and even clinicians. They can make the right decision for a patient without having to worry about how it will affect the bottom line.

So how do you know if you are burned out? If you are feeling more and more exhausted, find yourself feeling negative and cynical about work, or are mentally distancing yourself from your work, you are probably at risk. A nice online burnout questionnaire put together by the American Medical Association is found at *www.surveymonkey.com/r/WHPQWTJ*. It can be used to quantify your level of burnout. If you score highly on that, please consider meeting with a mental health professional.

As you prepare to enter your career, be aware of the existence of burnout and its prevalence among doctors. I have watched many people die during my career. None of them ever said on their deathbed that they wished they had spent more time at work. Maintain the relationships, habits, and outside interests that will allow you to overcome burnout. Increase your personal resilience whenever possible. Avoid and/or work to change abusive work situations. Consider the impact of every professional decision on your career longevity. The choice that will allow you to practice longer will almost always lead to more happiness and even a better financial outcome in the long run. Take care of your finances. Eliminating financial concerns from your life will reduce the likelihood of burnout, and facilitate solutions when it occurs.

MAIN IDEAS

- Burnout is common among physicians and can contribute to physician suicide.

- Financial planning can provide numerous burnout-reducing options.

ADDITIONAL RESOURCES

- **Blog Post:** Avoiding Burnout
  www.whitecoatinvestor.com/avoiding-burnout/

- **Blog Post:** Using a Venn-Diagram to Decrease Burnout
  www.whitecoatinvestor.com/using-a-venn-diagram-to-decrease-burnout/

- **Podcast:** #46 Physician Burnout with the Happy Philosopher
  www.whitecoatinvestor.com/physician-burnout-happy-philosopher-podcast-46/

- **Website:** The Physician Philosopher
  thephysicianphilosopher.com/

- **Resource:** Physician Life Coaching Services
  www.whitecoatinvestor.com/coaching

CHAPTER TWELVE

HOW TO CHOOSE A RESIDENCY PROGRAM

To be honest, there are only a few important financial decisions that one makes during medical or dental school. Obviously, choosing a specialty is the most important of those. A more minor decision involves choosing a residency program. For those students who are not at the very top of their class but still interested in a very competitive specialty, this might not even feel like a choice. Given the nature of the match, this decision will always be somewhat out of your control. But for the vast majority of medical students, and a significant percentage of top dental students interested in specializing, residency selection is mostly up to you. You get to choose which programs to apply to, you get to choose which interviews to attend, and you get to determine your rank list. That rank list really matters. In 2020, among graduating students from US MD schools applying for the first time, 46% matched at their first choice, 15% at their second choice, 9% at their third choice, and 6% at their fourth choice. Only 17% matched below their 4th choice.[33]

Obviously, you can only rank programs that you interviewed at, so some portion of that 46% did not actually end up going to the program that was their first choice when the process started, but it still stands to reason that a large percentage of students are able to choose their own residency program. The more competitive you are as an applicant, and the less competitive your chosen specialty, the more control you have over your residency program selection. So let me give you some advice about this decision you will face. Some of that advice will be financial, but most of it is not.

Remember that not matching is a financial catastrophe. So as important as it may be for you to go to one of your top choices, it is far more important, from a financial perspective, that you match somewhere. Here are some steps you can take to increase the odds of matching at a program in your chosen specialty.

First, have a realistic view of your competitiveness as an applicant. Know where you stack up in your class rank and with your board scores, at least for USMLE Step 2 since Step 1 scores will not be reported after 2021. Another really important factor is your grades in rotations in your chosen specialty. If ever there is a time to show up early, stay late, and really shine, it is during those rotations, both at your institution and away. Have an open and honest conversation with your faculty advisor, and if you are lucky enough to have one at your institution, with the residency program director in your chosen specialty, about your own competitiveness. Make sure you also understand the competitiveness of your specialty. I suspect many unmatched graduates overestimated their own competitiveness while underestimating the competitiveness of their specialty. If you are applying for the second time or from a Caribbean school, you are by definition not a competitive applicant. That really cannot be said about a DO applicant any more, but a DO is still slightly less competitive than an MD degree.

Second, decide how many programs to apply to. There is a financial cost to applying, but it pales in comparison to the cost of interviewing, much less the cost of not matching—although that may be changing given the virtual interviewing experience people are having in the 2020–2021 cycle during the COVID-19 pandemic. Err on the high side. If you get "too many" interviews, you can always turn them down. You can apply to up to 10 programs for just $99. Programs 11–20 cost $16 each. Programs 21–30 cost $20 each. Each program above 30 costs $26 each. Thus, your application cost would be:

MD Match Application Costs	
# of Programs	Total Cost
10	$99
20	$249
30	$439
50	$959
100	$2259

While \$2,259 is a lot of money to a medical student, it is not much compared to the cost of not matching. Losing one year of attending physician earnings is likely worth \$200,000 or more, depending on specialty. If you are a less than competitive applicant interested in a competitive specialty, 50–100 programs are not too many to apply to. In fact, in a few specialties, it is routine to apply to all of the programs. Talk to your faculty advisor and students from the class above you that went into that specialty for specific information.

Third, most medical students do not apply to 100+ programs. So they must choose the programs to which they will apply. For them, the rank list process begins with this step. You cannot rank a program to which you never applied. Obviously, apply to the programs you find most attractive. In every specialty, there are programs with a top-notch reputation. Apply to a few of these if they are in geographic locations that you would be willing to live in. Apply to all of the programs in your preferred geographic areas. Then be sure to apply to at least a few programs that would be considered less competitive to get into, whether due to reputation, the quality of education, or their geographic location. I cannot tell you how many students were glad they applied to "back-up programs" when they ended up overestimating their competitiveness and only received interviews at those back-up programs. Go ahead and start making your rank list now. Yes, it will change once you go on your interviews, but probably not as much as you think. This list can help guide you when applying and when accepting interviews.

Fourth, the next step of the process, receiving invitations to interview from the programs, is not completely out of your control either. The program directors are very much aware that you are applying to multiple programs— dozens of them in the competitive specialties. They do not want to waste their time interviewing people who are unlikely to rank them high just like you do not want to waste your time interviewing at your 20th choice. But just as you want to ensure that you match, they want to ensure that they fill their program. Yes, they want the best applicants, but they also want applicants who are very interested in their program. So consider sending your top two or three programs an email or a letter to let them know how interested you are. You can do this before the interview invitations start coming out, or only if you do not receive an invitation to your top programs. You might be surprised how often one of these letters results in an interview invitation. Even better, arrange to rotate at your top choice programs. That usually provides you an automatic interview, but remember that in this situation you are basically interviewing all month, so be on your very best behavior.

Fifth, now the interview invitations are starting to roll in and you will need to start scheduling interviews. Unfortunately, the least competitive programs tend to send out their invitations first, and those interview slots, especially on your preferred days, are limited. Thus, you cannot simply wait until you get all of your invitations and then choose which ones to accept. Start scheduling interviews as you receive invitations. If you receive more invitations than you can actually attend, be grateful. Cancel the one you are less interested in and schedule the latest invite on that day. If you have limited the geographic area that you applied to, it will be much easier to line up your interviews in a cost-effective way. If there are two geographic areas you have applied to, consider lining up the interviews in one area in December and the other in January. For instance, I applied in the West as well as Northern states. In December I went on a road trip. Starting in Minneapolis and finishing in Maine, I interviewed at a different program nearly every day. While I probably went to too many interviews (19 for the regular match), once I had them lined up in a row, there was little point in canceling one since I would be driving through that city that day anyway! The interviews out West were much cheaper for me to do two or three at a time, so I did those in January and February. Group your interviews as much as possible, perhaps 4–6 interviews per group, each group in one geographic area. Interview invitations roll in at random times. Keep your calendar on you so you can respond quickly to invitations and get your desired interview date, as well as rearrange other interviews as quickly as possible.

Consider scheduling the interviews at your top choices relatively late in the Winter. You will be a more polished interviewee and know better what you are looking for. Plus, you will still be top of mind when the program makes its rank list. Interviews are expensive compared to applications, so do what you can to minimize the cost. Combine trips whenever possible. Drive to interviews if you possibly can. While it will cost you a little gas money, you will save airfare and the costs of a rental car or public transportation. Sleep on the couches and spare beds of friends, friends of friends, family, prior graduates of your school, and if possible, residents in the program. Just remember that every single moment you are interacting with a resident or faculty member of the program is part of your interview. Finally, make sure you treat the seemingly low-ranking program coordinator like a king or queen. That person has a lot of influence on whether you match there.

Check with your school and alumni office to see if they have a hosting program. Many do. These programs consist of graduates from prior years who will open their homes to you when you come to interview. Often they are residents in another program at the hospital, but sometimes attendings participate as well. One new resource for this can be found at *www.swapandsnooze.com*, a free service where medical students and residents host and are hosted across the country.

Take some cheap food with you. Oatmeal packets can provide you breakfast if the program does not, and it is usually easy to get some hot water even in the sparsest of hotel rooms or short-term rentals. If possible, try to make the resident dinner the night before. It is a great opportunity to meet residents as they really are, but just as importantly, it is a great meal at a particularly good price! Just remember that the dinner is part of the interview. Those residents are often members of the match committee at the program. You can bring some pre-made food for lunches and dinners on days you do not have interviews or resident dinners too.

Find some reasonably conservative, business-like clothing. One suit is plenty for guys, but get another shirt and tie, just in case you spill something. A couple of outfits are probably fine for the ladies too. The only person who knows you wore that outfit two days ago at another program (because they also interviewed there) does not have any influence over whether you match at this program. Nobody cares if it is a $200 suit or a $1,000 suit as long as it is presentable.

I have learned other tips from more recent graduates. For example, one recommended scheduling as many of your interview flights as possible on Southwest Airlines. Their no-cost change policy allows you to reschedule and rearrange interviews without as much expense. In fact, you might start using a credit card that gives you airline miles during medical school. Then when it comes time to interview, you can purchase many of your flights with miles instead of cash. A sign-on bonus alone may pay for an entire flight.

Be frugal, but not so cheap that it costs you the financial catastrophe of not matching. The costs can be covered with money that you earn as an MS4, by taking out a little more in student loans that year, with a special private loan (usually at a higher interest rate), or in a worst-case but common scenario, put on credit cards. If you go this route, try to get new credit cards with 12-month 0% introductory offers, and prioritize paying them off as a new intern before they start generating interest.

Once you have completed your interviews, it is time to finalize your rank list. Make a spreadsheet of all the programs on the Y-axis and all of the factors that matter to you and your significant other on the X-axis. After careful thought, finalize your rank list and let the top program or two know that they are ranked very highly on your list. It cannot hurt. Let me give you some advice about the most important factors.

In my opinion, the most important factor is the people in the program, both faculty and residents. You want a good fit here. You will be working with these people 80 hours a week for the next 3–5 years. Make sure you like them. They will continue to attract people like them in the coming years. If you are single and most of the residents in the program are married with children, you may not fit in so well. If you are into hiking and mountain biking, matching in a big city where the residents spend their limited spare time clubbing or shopping may be a mismatch.

Next, make sure the quality of the education is sufficient for your needs. If the program is on probation, if procedure counts are too low to develop expertise, or if graduates are having trouble passing their board exams, you probably want to steer clear. The main purpose of residency is to become a fantastic doctor. How easy will it be to do that in this program? In addition, make sure the program meets your unique needs and interests. Make sure that there is sufficient exposure to the subspecialties, procedures, and diseases in which you have the most interest.

Perhaps the next most important factor is location. Some of us are big city people. We prefer to be around a diverse population with hundreds of restaurants, professional sports teams, and cultural opportunities. Others of us prefer a smaller city or even a more rural location. If possible, try to train in a city that is similar to where you will live later, as the population and pathology will be similar. If you are married or have a serious partner, their input will also be very important on this topic, and perhaps even more important than yours. Significant others of residents are often described as "functionally single" during the training years, and my wife and I can certainly relate. She still has reunions with the very close friends she made in Tucson that I barely know. The people I grew to know well during those years all seemed to work in the hospital for some reason. Do not underestimate the value of doing your residency in a place where your partner has connections and community. This can be a tremendous asset at a stressful time for a relationship as it can alleviate the pressure on the resident when their partner has a job and friends to keep them busy during those long call shifts.

So consider these questions for your significant other:

> Can they get a job there?
>
> Can they study what they wish to study in this location?
>
> Do they already have friends there (or are they particularly adept at making new ones)?
>
> Do they already have family in the city?

If you already have or are planning to have children during residency, consider your childcare options in each possible residency location. Childcare can be very expensive, and not necessarily available at the times that resident physicians are working. They may not open early enough to allow you to start rounding at 5 a.m., much less stay open until you get off at 8 p.m. Some hospitals provide childcare, find out if yours is one of them. Supportive family in the area is another great option that can be particularly useful for evening, weekend, holiday, and overnight childcare.

If you are entering the couples match, your geographic choices will be even more constrained (and your match process much more competitive). There is an additional factor that should be considered as far as location, and that is the cost of living. A resident typically earns $50,000–$60,000 per year, about the median US household income. There is a little bit of a variation in salary and benefits from one program to another, but it pales in comparison to the cost of living. You will make about $60,000 a year no matter where you go. That money will go much further in Indianapolis or Lawton, Oklahoma than it will in San Francisco or Manhattan. This will have a significant impact on your ability to start building wealth by paying off debt, saving up an emergency fund or a down payment, and even starting to invest for retirement or college during residency. But most importantly, it will have a massive effect on your lifestyle—how nice of a home you will live in, what you will drive, how you will vacation, what you can buy, and how often you can go out. This is especially important if you will have dependents during residency. While finances should not be the most important factor in residency selection, I would encourage you to at least have a line for cost of living on your spreadsheet.

Some medical students have asked me how much weight they should place on salary, health insurance, available retirement plans, and similar benefits. My response? Almost none. The options are just too similar between medical residency programs. While it is great if they will offer you a bit of a 401(k) match and a higher salary, it would not change my rank list in any significant way. With careful financial management, you can make up for any differences in your first month as an attending physician. You can save dramatically more money on an attending salary than a resident salary. Be smart about money, but do not try to get rich as a resident. That can wait for the attending years. Concentrate on becoming a great doctor and the money will come.

Most of the above information applies to dentists as well as physicians. However, due to the financial nature of dental residencies, dentists will need to give a little more weight to the financial implications of their residency choice, whether a GPR/AEGD residency or one of the specialties. Salary/stipend, cost of tuition, and cost of living should all be factored more heavily than it would be for a graduating medical student. Given that the cost of attendance can vary by $100,000 or more per year of residency, skew your applications, interviews, and final rank list toward the programs that charge less and/or pay more. Obviously, you want to make sure you will be getting the education you need, and of course you have to actually get into the program, but doubling or tripling your student loan debt during residency is going to have a severe impact on your future financial life.

While financial considerations should not be highly weighted by anyone during the residency selection process, they cannot be ignored completely, especially for dental specialists. Good luck in the match!

MAIN IDEAS

- Primary considerations with residency selection should be fit with the faculty and other residents and the quality of the education.

- Location of the residency is another major factor with significant financial ramifications.

- There are many ways to save money while still applying and interviewing broadly enough to ensure you match.

ADDITIONAL RESOURCES

- **Blog Post:** Choosing a Residency: What Goes into a Rank List
  www.kevinmd.com/blog/2014/03/choosing-perfect-residency-rank-list.html

- **Blog Post:** 10 Ways to Reduce Residency Interview Expenses
  www.whitecoatinvestor.com/10-ways-to-minimize-residency-interview-expenses/

- **Blog Post:** Spend Less and Interview More
  www.whitecoatinvestor.com/residency-interviews-spend-less-and-interview-more/

- **Blog Post:** Financial Survival as a Resident
  www.whitecoatinvestor.com/financial-survival-as-a-resident/

- **Blog Post:** How to Live like a Resident as a Resident
  www.whitecoatinvestor.com/how-to-live-like-a-resident-as-a-resident/

CHAPTER THIRTEEN

WHY A DENTIST SHOULD NOT BE AFRAID TO OPEN A PRACTICE

Over the last 20 years, fewer and fewer physicians own their own jobs. From 2001 to 2016, the percentage of physician owners decreased from 61% to 47%.[34] Practice owners are selling their practices to hospitals and taking on a job as an employee. Solo practice owners are now incredibly rare and almost no new residency graduates are opening their own practice. Much of this is due to the burden of compliance with government mandates, aside from the difficulties inherent in running your own business. This trend also exists but is not nearly as profound among dentists. Historically, 80% of dentists became sole proprietors, with most of the rest in multi-dentist partnerships. Those numbers are both certainly lower now, although the data is somewhat difficult to find.

From 2005 to 2015, the percentage of dentists who owned their practice declined from 84% to 80%. The drop is even more profound among dentists under 35, where the decrease went from 44% to 38%. Although nobody knows exactly why this is happening, the causes are generally thought to be rising student debt, the emergence of corporate dentistry, and shifting work-life balance preferences. Some have speculated that it is due, at least in part, to a rising percentage of female dentists. However, this seems unlikely to be the most important factor given that the percentage of women who own their own practice actually rose slightly during that time period, and the percentage of women in dentistry only rose from 20% to 29% over that decade.[35]

However, as you can see from the data I cited in a previous chapter, practice owners generally make more money than employees. I will reproduce the table again here for your convenience.[36]

Type of Dentist	Average	1st Quartile	Median	3rd Quartile
General Practitioners				
All Owners	$201,860	$120,000	$175,000	$250,000
Solo	$187,810	$110,000	$158,000	$240,000
Nonsolo	$235,720	$142,500	$200,000	$300,000
Employed	$160,110	$95,000	$150,000	$191,000
All General Practitioners	**$190,440**	**$110,000**	**$160,000**	**$250,000**
Specialists				
All Owners	$356,670	$200,000	$300,000	$475,000
Solo	$340,250	$180,000	$300,000	$450,000
Nonsolo	$378,230	$216,000	$350,000	$500,000
Employed	$257,280	$165,000	$220,000	$344,000
All Specialists	**$330,180**	**$180,000**	**$280,000**	**$406,000**
All Dentists				
All Owners	$233,840	$120,000	$200,000	$300,000
Solo	$214,190	$120,000	$175,000	$275,000
Nonsolo	$275,240	$150,000	$250,000	$360,000
Employed	$184,790	$108,000	$160,000	$230,000
All Dentists	**$220,950**	**$120,000**	**$180,000**	**$280,000**

The median owner makes 17% more money. Among more successful dentists (3rd quartile), that number increases to 31%. The number is likely even higher among the most successful dentists. A small percentage of dentists earns more than $500,000 per year, or even more than $1 million. I assure you that these doctors are all owners of their practices. In fact, your ability to generate a high income will likely have more to do with your ability to run a business in an intelligent and efficient way than your technical skill or bedside manner. Employees are starting out behind because, over the long run, it does not make sense to pay an employee exactly what the employee is worth. The employee must generate enough in revenue to cover her own pay and benefits, and leave something left over for the business owner. It does not make sense to hire employees that cost you more than they bring in.

Being an employee dentist certainly has some conveniences—no hassles of ownership, a steady income, and a relatively easy ability to move from one job to another or even across the country. But it comes at a cost. Not only do you lose control and flexibility, but you make less money. That would be fine if the cost of becoming a dentist were not so high. Certainly $150,000 per year provides a pretty nice lifestyle. But if you have $600,000 in student loans to pay off, $150,000 is not going to cut it. The debt-to-income ratio is simply too high, unless that job also qualifies for Public Service Loan Forgiveness (PSLF).

Many graduating dentists are afraid to become practice owners these days. While the normal jitters will always apply ("I do not know how to run a business, I am not even sure I know how to be a good dentist yet"), many of these dentists are deterred by their student loan burdens from taking on the risks and costs of opening or buying a practice of their own. Ownership will never be right for all dentists, but I want to reassure you that just having a high student loan burden should not be a reason to avoid owning a practice. In fact, I would argue that the higher your student loans, the more you need to own your job. You simply need a higher income to pay them off.

It can be scary to come out of dental school with $500,000 in student loans, buy a house with a $500,000 mortgage, and then borrow another $500,000–$1 million to buy or start a practice, especially when you might only earn $150,000–$200,000 that first year. As you know from an earlier chapter, you do not get a pass on math just because you have chosen to become a dentist or because you have chosen to buy a practice. However, I have three recommendations that should help.

First, do not buy the $500,000 house. In fact, maybe do not buy a house at all for a while. I tell physicians to "Live like a Resident" for a while once they enter practice. If you can "Live like a Dental Student" for a while you will be much better off financially. While you do not want to be "house-poor" or "practice-poor," the practice is likely a far better investment in the long run. If you do buy a house, perhaps you can buy it primarily as an investment property, turning it into an additional source of income in a few years when you are in a better financial position.

Second, work really hard. You will never be so excited about your career as the first few years out of school, especially when the money from working is so useful. Consider offering evening and weekend hours. Early morning hours can also be very attractive. One dentist who reviewed this book starts the day at 7 a.m. and finds that the first two hours of the day are always the busiest. This will distinguish you from surrounding practices and help you to grow faster. If you have free time during the day, spend it marketing, both online and in person. Perhaps you can even maintain a second job as an associate for a while, but carefully review the contract first to ensure there will not be a problem with a non-compete or non-solicitation clause.

Third, it is okay to start small and have room to grow. You can literally double the production of an old declining practice in the first year just by updating the technology and providing new services.

Remember that the practice loan is not the same thing as your student loans. First, the interest may be deductible, lowering the after-tax cost of the loan. More importantly, you received something for the money that can later be sold. There is nothing you can sell to get your student loan money back. It is like you took a mortgage out on your brain and have to hope nobody forecloses on it! The practice, its real estate, and its equipment all have some value, so while your debt-to-income ratio increased, your net worth did not change when you bought the practice.

You might also consider a sweat equity type buy-in if you are planning to take over another dentist's practice in a few years. This is common among physician partnerships. The doctor basically works for less than they are generating for a few years, and are paid with equity in the practice. Just make sure the agreement is fair to all parties. The practice owner may even be willing to finance your purchase of the practice.

It will be easier for you to pay off your loans and build wealth on $175,000 than on $150,000, but the real benefit, especially for someone who works hard to build a great business, comes in a few more years when you are earning $300,000 or more per year instead of that same old $150,000 you would still be making as an associate. Even after-tax, an extra $100,000 or more a year goes a long way toward wiping out your student loans, practice loan, and mortgage.

It will involve a lot more work and stress, especially in the short term, to be a practice owner. In the long run, you will benefit from more income, more tax deductions, and more control, all while building a valuable asset that can be sold to help fund your retirement. Many older dentists will tell you, "There is no way I would go into dentistry if I could not work for myself." Listen to them. A decade from now you will appreciate the income, but you will really love controlling your own destiny.

MAIN IDEAS

- Almost all of the highest earners in dentistry are practice owners, not employees.

- A high dental school loan burden may require you to eventually own your own practice.

- Having control over your professional life by owning your practice is so valuable that many dentists say they would not go into dentistry again if they were not able to do so.

ADDITIONAL RESOURCES

- **Blog Post:** Ownership Has Its Privileges
  www.whitecoatinvestor.com/ownership-has-its-privileges/

- **Article:** Ready to Own Your Own Dental Office? It Isn't for Everyone
  www.dentalentrepreneur.com/808-2/

- **Website:** Dentaltown
  www.dentaltown.com/

PART TWO

PART TWO

MANAGING FINANCES DURING RESIDENCY

Nearly all medical students and some dental students reading this book will soon become residents. Thinking about residency can be intimidating due to the stress and many hours of hard work involved. But it is also exciting to finally start practicing as an apprentice doctor. Despite its rigors and low pay, to this day my favorite job that I ever had was being a resident. Resident doctors do not have a lot of time for much of anything beyond learning their trade, but since this training period can last anywhere from one to seven years, you cannot simply ignore money the whole time and expect to be financially successful.

There are a few financial tasks to do and a few unique opportunities to take advantage of during residency. Part two of this book is going to go through them one by one. We will discuss homeownership, including a lengthy discussion of the oft-debated "Rent versus Buy" question. I will also teach you the best ways to manage your student loans. We will discuss the ways you can get started investing and we will talk about critical types of insurance, including disability and life insurance. Armed with this information, you will easily move into the early years of your residency confident that you are not making any significant financial mistakes. This will allow you to spend your time and energy on becoming a proficient, compassionate doctor.

CHAPTER FOURTEEN

WHY RENTING COULD ACTUALLY SAVE YOU MONEY

Medical and dental students, and particularly their partners, have a strange burning desire to become homeowners. Perhaps it exists among most Americans in their twenties and I only notice it among professional students, but I find it to be a strange phenomenon. Perhaps it is a result of heavy marketing by the real estate agent and mortgage lending industries. Maybe it is a result of misguided advice from older generations. Perhaps it is a gradual molding over the decades of "The American Dream" from starting a business from scratch to owning a home. Perhaps it is that people feel parents should own a home to provide a stable environment for their children. Whatever it is, there is no doubt that almost every medical and dental student, particularly if they are married, wants to buy a home. So what is the problem? Well, most of the time it is not the right financial move to buy before completing training. These graduating students also will not realize until later that it really did not provide any substantial non-monetary benefits.

Lots of people mistakenly think that "renting is throwing money away." That is absolutely not true. Renting is exchanging money for a place to live. You exchange money for food to eat and entertainment to watch all the time, but do not view that as throwing money away. Paying for housing is no different.

I have been advising graduating students for over a decade not to buy a home until they are in a stable personal and employment situation, meaning after residency. Most of them do not listen. I literally cannot talk them out of losing thousands or even tens of thousands of dollars on average. Part of the difficulty of taking that advice is that they do not ALL lose money. Perhaps one-third of those who buy for a three-year residency actually come out ahead from buying. That number probably rises to 50% for those who buy for a five-year period. Obviously, if you spend seven years in one location doing a neurosurgery residency the odds may actually be in your favor.

What determines whether you will be in the 33–50% of typical residents that make money? While smart decisions about purchasing, maintaining, and upgrading can help, the primary factor that determines whether you make money on such a short-term home purchase is completely out of your control—appreciation. The home simply has to appreciate enough to overcome the substantial costs of buying and selling. It typically will not do so during a three to four-year stint in school or residency. On average you will lose money. If you talk to financially savvy doctors, even those who made money owning a home during residency, most will acknowledge it was a mistake and they just got lucky.

Luckily, the realization of that mistake is generally accompanied by a substantial rise in income, such that the mistake can easily be afforded. However, as the average student loan burden rises, along with downward stress on doctor incomes, optimizing your finances is becoming more and more important, and this is an easy decision to optimize. How can you optimize it? It is as easy as renting your primary residence until such a time as your personal and professional situation is stable and looks to remain that way for the next 5–10+ years.

Now do not get me wrong. I am a big fan of ownership in general. Being an owner with your investments (i.e. stocks and real estate) generally pays off a lot better than not being an owner (i.e. cash and bonds). I also like seeing doctors own their jobs as sole proprietors or partners as it gives them more flexibility, control, and income. I am also a big fan of home ownership and currently own my home. But as the Preacher says in Ecclesiastes, for everything there is a season, and a time for every activity.[37] Medical school and residency are not the ideal time to be a homeowner.

Let me give you a couple of examples from my own life of times I bought a home when I really should not have. The first one was in medical school. We bought a little condo on a bus line 10 minutes away from the school. It cost us $80,000. The mortgage payment alone was ⅔ of my HPSP stipend, and that is not counting the mandatory HOA fee. When we left for residency, we put it up for sale. It took several months to sell. Meanwhile, we were paying rent in the new place and still paying the mortgage on an empty condo. We sold it for $83,000. We won, right? We sold it for more than we bought it for and should be happy, no? Well, not really. Once you take into consideration the transaction costs (including it sitting empty for two months at the end), of approximately 5% to get in and 10% to get out, we really needed that property to appreciate about 15% to break even. Since it only appreciated about 4% over those four years, we came out behind. Especially when we later learned that comparable places were renting for even less than our mortgage!

The second example was when I was in the military. I had a four-year active duty obligation after residency, and we figured we would spend it all in the same place. (That did end up happening, but we nearly ended up changing duty station 2–3 years into the job.) So we bought an affordable townhome. This was in 2006, and those who know financial history know what came next. Four years later, we could not find a buyer at any sort of reasonable price, even for one-third less than we had paid for it (at which price it would be a fantastic rental property). We tried to sell it for over a year without success before finally giving up and putting a renter in there for four more years. We eventually sold it nine years after purchasing for 12% less than we paid for it back in 2006.

I have had countless doctors confirm similar experiences with houses they bought in residency. They often move to a different city for their post-residency job and even if they do not, they really do not want to live in the house they could afford as a resident for very long. Sometimes they have trouble selling the place and end up with two mortgages for a while. Sometimes they end up selling for a loss. Sometimes they put a renter in there and end up with a cash flow negative property that they try to manage from out-of-state. Even those for whom it worked out well generally admit, "I just got lucky, it was not a great decision a priori and I would not do it again."

You may have seen statistics showing that, for the typical American, the value of their home is a significant portion of their wealth. The problem is that you do not hear the countering statistic that the typical American did not really build any significant amount of wealth. If you look at the hard numbers, you will quickly decide that you do not want to be typical in this regard. The median American between 65 and 74 has just $126,000 saved for retirement. This provides a monthly income of approximately $420. Add $1,000–$2,000 of monthly Social Security income to that and you can see what that typical American retires on. The median net worth of someone in that age group is $224,000. Most of the remainder of that net worth is the value of their home equity. So it is true that a big chunk of their net worth comes from owning their home. But it certainly did not make them wealthy.

In fact, for many of them, the house kept them from building wealth due to the cost of interest, property taxes, insurance, maintenance, and furnishings. That is not even considering the effect of trying to keep up with the Joneses in their too-expensive neighborhood. They became house poor. This often happens to students and residents who buy houses. Admittedly doctors generally buy more expensive houses than the typical American, but a doctor who becomes financially independent certainly does not have half their net worth tied up in their house. The house more likely makes up < 20% of their net worth, and usually less than 10%. If you become successful, the value of your house will not be a major part of your financial life.

Some may be offered a "rent to buy" option. While every contract is different, these are rarely a great deal for the tenant/prospective owner. Basically, you get overcharged rent while some tiny portion of it goes toward a potential discount you may get down the road if you actually buy the house. If you do not end up buying the house, you lose all of that "equity" you paid for through the overpriced rent.

Let us conclude this chapter with a discussion of the top 10 reasons a resident (and even more so a student) should not buy their home. Honestly, I doubt any of this will talk you out of buying a house. But I hope you would at least consider renting a home, as it really should be the default option for a short time period like residency.

10 REASONS A RESIDENT SHOULD NOT BUY A HOME

1 – You Do Not Have a Down Payment

You can buy a home with less than a standard down payment, or in many cases with no down payment at all. However, there are a few benefits to putting down a standard 20% down payment. You will have:

- More lenders to choose from,
- A lower interest rate,

- Lower fees,

- No private mortgage insurance (PMI),

- An easier time passing underwriting,

- A smaller mortgage on which interest is calculated, and

- More of a safety buffer in the event the home depreciates.

In addition, the act of saving up a down payment is useful as it teaches you to budget and to understand just how much home you can really afford while still reaching your other financial goals.

One thing most graduating professional students do not have, however, is a lot of cash. Not only do they have several hundred thousand dollars in student loans, but they likely have a car debt, some credit card debt, and maybe even some debt from the interview and moving processes. They do not have an extra $20,000–$100,000 sitting around to function as a real down payment. If you stay there for a long time, buying a home with less than 20% down can certainly work out just fine. There are even special doctor loans that offer lower down payments without requiring private mortgage insurance. You can find out who offers these in your state at *www.whitecoatinvestor.com/mortgage*. Despite these, it is still a bad idea for most residents to buy a house. Just because someone will lend you money, does not mean you should take it. Lenders only care that you have enough income to make the payments. The underwriting process does not ensure that you have enough income to make the payments and reach your other financial goals.

2 – You Do Not Have Any Income

Besides a down payment, the other thing a resident needs to get a conventional mortgage is proven income. There are lenders willing to lend you money without a down payment or proven income, but your options will be more limited, which will result in more hassle, a higher interest rate, and higher fees. The typical process is to get the job first, save up some money, prove your ability to make money in the future, and then buy a house a few months or a few years later. Buying during residency shortcuts this process, and that has consequences.

3 – You Have Tons of Debt Already

Honestly, a typical resident with a $200,000–$300,000 student loan burden already has more debt than can be afforded on a resident salary. It does not seem like a wise time to add on more, especially for something that functions at least as much as a liability as an asset.

4 – Residency Is Only Three to Five Years Long

This is the biggest reason why residents should not buy a home. Historically, homes appreciate at about the rate of inflation. Perhaps slightly more, but more or less you should expect average appreciation over many years to work out to about 2–4%. Obviously, some areas will appreciate faster while others will appreciate more slowly, not at all, or even depreciate. However, knowing that in advance requires a functioning crystal ball, which neither you nor I have. But in order to break even, you really need that property to appreciate about 15% while you are in it. That is unlikely to happen by the three-year mark. It is more likely at the five-year mark, but even then it is still mostly a coin flip. Since most residents are in that home only three to five years, the majority of them do not see enough appreciation to come out ahead. Everybody thinks they are an exception to this rule of thumb. A few people are exceptions (such as those living in the same house for medical school and residency or being married to a high earner whose job will keep you anchored there after residency), but you probably are not one of them.

5 – You Can Rent a House

Part of the issue with renting is the image people have in their mind. They think renting means apartment living and after four years of undergraduate and four years of medical or dental school, they are sick of apartment living. They want four bedrooms, they want more space, and they want a backyard for the kids or a dog. What they may not realize, however, is that they can rent a house nearly as easily as they can rent an apartment in most cities large enough to have residency programs. There are plenty of real estate investors who own single-family homes and want to rent them out. These exist in poor neighborhoods, median neighborhoods, and the fanciest neighborhoods in town. They would be thrilled to rent to resident physicians, and may even offer a rent discount in exchange for a multi-year contract. A reliable person with a reliable income who is going to stay for three to five years? That is a pretty easy rental decision. A 30-second online search shows that right now in my city there are about 1800 places for rent. About 200 of them are single-family homes of varying sizes and prices. Occasionally there will be a situation where a resident literally cannot find what they need to live in and will be forced to buy, but that is a pretty rare situation. You do not have to rent an apartment in most cities with residency programs.

6 – New Home Owners Underestimate the Cost of Homeownership

Most residents that buy a home are doing so for the first time and routinely underestimate the costs of homeownership. They might even be so ignorant as to think that if the mortgage is less than comparable rent that they will come out ahead. An experienced real estate investor knows that approximately 45% of what is collected as rent will go toward non-mortgage costs. So of course the landlord must charge more in rent than the mortgage payment in order to have a profitable investment. Think of all the other costs of homeownership:

> Property Taxes
>
> Insurance
>
> Maintenance
>
> Upgrades
>
> Snow Removal
>
> Lawn Care
>
> Tools
>
> Utilities (Electric, Gas, Water, Wastewater, Garbage)

This list ignores the vacancies and management costs that a landlord would also be dealing with. Most graduating medical students do not own a broom, much less a lawnmower, but if they buy a house with a lawn, they are going to need both of those items. The cost will not be insignificant on a resident income.

7 – You Will Not Live in That Home as an Attending

A lot of residents justify their home purchase with the thought that they will stay in that home as an attending. While that is entirely possible, it is unlikely.

First, a large percentage of docs leave town to practice somewhere else after residency. What are the odds that the best job for you is in the same town as your residency? Probably not very high.

Second, it would be very unusual for someone that makes $250,000 or more to be happy in the same home a resident could afford on an income of $50,000 for very long. I counsel graduating residents to try to live like a resident for a while to get themselves set up on a solid financial footing, but the truth is that almost everyone upgrades their lifestyle at least a little upon residency graduation. That 1400 square foot bungalow that seemed like a mansion compared to the 500 square foot apartment you had as a med student is not going to seem adequate when those attending-size paychecks start rolling in.

8 – Home Maintenance Costs Either Time or Money

When you rent, much of your home maintenance will be taken care of by the landlord. Fixing broken appliances, repairing leaky roofs or windows, cutting the lawn, or removing snow all costs either time or money, neither of which is abundant for a resident. Do you really want to spend your only days off this month shopping for and installing a new dishwasher? The less of this you have to worry about, the more time you can spend learning medicine and the more money you can use to stabilize your financial future. Aside from the maintenance, just buying and selling a home can be pretty stressful. Do you really need that stress between medical school and residency, or between residency and your first job?

9 – Residents Do Not Get a Tax Break for Owning a Home

Lots of realtors and mortgage agents like to sell homeownership as "The American Dream." Their second favorite sales angle is to convince you that you will lower your taxes by becoming a homeowner. However, the likelihood of that happening in any significant way as a resident is quite low. In 2021, a couple filing Married Filing Jointly (MFJ) has a standard deduction of $25,100. That means until you have at least $25,100 in itemized deductions including charitable gifts, mortgage interest, and taxes (including up to $10,000 in state income taxes and property taxes), none of it is really deductible. Even if you manage to come up with a few thousand more than $25,100, really only the amount above and beyond that is an additional deduction you received for buying the house.

This is not going to create a tax break for most residents. They just do not spend more than that on anything that becomes an itemized deduction. If you are single, the bar is lower, but it is still $12,400 before anything is really deductible. Part of the reason you may wish to own a home as an attending is the tax benefits, but most residents are not going to see any of those. Residents just cannot afford a big enough house that mortgage interest and property taxes are more than the standard deduction. At 3% interest, $20,000 in mortgage interest would suggest a mortgage of almost $700,000—utter foolishness on a resident income!

10 – Budgeting Is Easier as a Renter

Living on a tight budget is not ever easy, but it is far easier to budget for a simple rent payment each month than it is to account for the myriad of variable expenses you will run into as a homeowner. As an attending, you replace an appliance out of your monthly earnings. As a resident, you would have to clean out your emergency fund to do the same thing. You can also project your housing costs upfront—exactly 36 months of rent for a three-year residency as opposed to who knows how many repairs you will have to do and how many months it will take you to sell when you move on to your attending job.

As I mentioned earlier, you can actually come out ahead buying during residency. It is not impossible to do so. But the odds are stacked against you. The longer the residency, the better your chances. It can also be helpful if you are married to a high earner, so perhaps you might see some tax benefits from the purchase. The increase in income as an attending can also make up for losing money on the residency house. But the default option should still be to rent until your personal and professional lives are stable. For most doctors, that time is after completion of residency and once you know you like your job and your job likes you. Until then, find something that meets your needs to rent. At least think about it.

MAIN IDEAS

- On average, it requires about five years to break even on a home purchase, but this can be highly variable. Some lose money despite owning longer and some people get lucky and come out ahead from owning for just a year or two.

- Since most residencies are three to five years long and very busy, most residents should rent their residence during their training.

ADDITIONAL RESOURCES

- **Resource:** New York Times Buy vs. Rent Calculator
  www.nytimes.com/interactive/2014/upshot/buy-rent-calculator.html

- **Blog Post:** The Doctor Mortgage Loan
  www.whitecoatinvestor.com/personal-finance/the-doctor-mortgage-loan/

- **Blog Post:** Physician Mortgage Loans for Other High-Income Professionals
  www.whitecoatinvestor.com/physician-mortgage-loans-for-other-high-income-professionals/

- **Resource:** Physician Mortgage Lenders
  www.whitecoatinvestor.com/mortgage

CHAPTER FIFTEEN

STUDENT LOAN MANAGEMENT DURING RESIDENCY

For the most part, nobody really gets wealthy during residency. I have long said that the most important year of your financial life is your first year out of training. If you can get that right, you can mess up almost anything else financially and still recover. However, there are several things that you can get wrong during residency that will really set you back in your financial journey. The first of these is not managing your student loans properly. It is unfortunate that most medical and dental schools provide little to no information about proper student loan management. Given the rapidly climbing nature of the average student loan burden, especially for the most indebted quartile of students, this lack of information becomes especially tragic. To make matters worse, in the last five years it has become even more complex to manage student loans properly.

In this chapter, I will provide the basic principles of proper student loan management in residency. However, some people are in such a complex situation that a book chapter by itself simply cannot meet their needs. If you are in that situation, know that this is a good place to spend a few hundred dollars and get some professional help with the most critical decisions. If you do not know who to trust, consider checking out the resources here:

Resource: Recommended Student Loan Advisors
www.whitecoatinvestor.com/student-loan-advice/

One might think that taking care of student loans would be simple. In fact, it used to be simple. Then the government got involved. Government programs have been very helpful for hundreds of thousands of doctors, but the potpourri of available programs has increased the complexity of management decisions by at least an order of magnitude. As it becomes more complex, more and more doctors do not manage their loans in an optimal manner. We will start with the easy decisions and move toward the more complex ones. First, we will discuss private student loans since their management is less complex. Then we will move on to federal student loans.

Loan Benefits	
Federal Loans	**Private Loans**
Lower rate during school	Lower rate after refinancing
Low IDR payments	$100 payments in residency
Eligible for employer and state payoff programs	Eligible for employer and state payoff programs
PSLF and IDR Forgiveness	Better customer service
Forgiven in event of death and permanent disability	Death and disability provisions vary by lender

PRIVATE STUDENT LOANS

Ideally, a medical or dental student does not have any private student loans. Private loans are not eligible for Income-Driven Repayment (IDR) programs or for the government forgiveness programs. They also generally carry higher interest rates. So when students do have private loans, it generally means they also have a massive federal student loan burden. Some International Medical Graduates (IMGs) are exceptions to this rule, since their school may not have qualified them to use the federal student loan system. Compared to managing federal student loans, managing private student loans is downright simple. Since no one is going to forgive them, and you have plenty of other loans to pay off with any potential future employer-based student loan repayment program, you can be sure that, barring death or permanent disability, you will be paying these loans off yourself.

You can get started at any time. Paying off a student loan with a 6–10% interest rate immediately eliminates the interest that you would be paying on that loan—which basically provides you a guaranteed after-tax return of 6–10% on that "investment." This should be very attractive given that for years the best rate of return you have been able to find on a guaranteed investment has been in the 1–2% range. There is essentially no justification for carrying that level of debt in order to invest money elsewhere. While it is not impossible to earn more than 6–10% investing, once you adjust for risk and taxes, it generally is not wise to even try. Just pay down the loans instead.

Student Loan Refinancing

Around the time of the Global Financial Crisis of 2007–2009, it became impossible to refinance student loans. Whatever you took out was what you had until you paid it off. Starting in 2011–2014, a few companies started popping up that were willing to refinance student loans again. It did not seem possible, nor fair, that you could get a mortgage at less than 3% but you could not get a student loan at less than 6–8%. By refinancing the loans, a borrower was able to reduce their interest rate by 1–4%. This could make a big difference on the loans that doctors were carrying around. 4% of a $300,000 loan is $12,000 a year that can go toward principal instead of interest. If payments stay the same after refinancing, the debt will be paid off years sooner with much less cumulative interest paid.

So it became a no-brainer for The White Coat Investor to partner with these companies to provide the best possible deals to our readers and listeners. You can find a current list here:

Resource: Recommended Student Loan Refinancing Companies
www.whitecoatinvestor.com/student-loan-refinancing

We negotiated for you to not only receive a much lower interest rate, saving you tens of thousands of dollars of interest over the course of the loan, but also to receive a cashback payment, usually consisting of several hundred dollars. Did you get that? Not only does it cost you nothing to apply and refinance, but you will actually be paid to do it. In fact, every time you refinance with a new company you will be paid a few hundred dollars to do it. So when it comes to private loans, you should refinance early and often.

As interest rates fluctuate and your credit score and debt-to-income ratios improve, you will qualify for better and better terms on your loan. It is not unusual at all for a doctor to have refinanced private loans three or four times before they are paid off. Now obviously we get paid too for connecting you to these companies, so of course we have a conflict of interest here. However, due to the extra cashback you would not get if you go directly to the companies, refinancing through these links is such a no-brainer for most docs that it seemed a disservice for me to not tell you about them in this section of the book.

The main benefit of refinancing your loans is the lower interest rate (although the cash bonus is nice). In order to get the lowest possible interest rate, you need to take on the most amount of risk. These lending companies take on two risks.

The first is interest rate risk. Interest rates fluctuate from month to month and year to year, sometimes quite severely. When a bank or other lender offers you a fixed-rate loan, the lender is running the risk that interest rates go up significantly early in the loan. Now instead of being able to lend that money out at a higher rate, they are stuck earning a much lower rate of return until you pay off the loan. If you will offer to run this risk for them, they will offer you a lower interest rate. This is called a variable interest rate loan. When interest rates rise, your payments go up. When interest rates fall, your payments go down. The risk is now on you. But on average, you will come out ahead using a variable rate loan. Think about it. If interest rates fall, your payments decrease. You win. If interest rates stay the same, you benefit from the lower interest rate you were offered. Again, you win. If interest rates go up just a little bit, or do not go up until the loan is almost paid off, you still win, since the benefit of the lower rate in the beginning of the loan more than makes up for the costs of the higher rate at the end.

The only time you lose with a variable interest rate loan is when rates go up a lot and do so early in the loan term. By taking out a fixed-rate loan, you are essentially buying an insurance policy against rates going up. Like any insurance policy, there is a cost. On average, paying someone else to run the risk for you is a losing proposition. It must be, or insurance companies would not exist. They must pay out less in benefits than they take in with premiums. The difference is used to pay their expenses and profits. So if you can afford to run interest rate risk, then do so. Calculate out the worst-case scenario on a variable rate loan. If you can afford it, take it. The risk probably will not show up. If you cannot afford to take that risk, then you will have to insure against it with a fixed-rate loan.

The second risk that lending companies take on is term risk. The longer you take to pay off your loans, the longer it will be before they can lend that money out to someone else (hopefully at a higher rate). Plus, a longer loan term increases the chance that you will default on the loan. Thus, if you are willing to commit to pay the debt off over a shorter time period, the lender is willing to offer you a lower interest rate. This is why 15-year mortgages come with lower interest rates than 30-year mortgages, all else being equal. If you will commit to paying off your loans within five years of completing your training, as I have already recommended to you, then you can qualify for the best rates that student loan refinancing companies will offer to you. Paying loans off quickly also reduces the interest rate risk that you would be running with a variable rate loan, since you will be exposed to the risks of a rapid rise in interest rates for a much shorter time period. If you want to pay as little interest as possible, apply for a five-year, variable-rate loan. Then pay extra on it whenever possible to be done even sooner.

Deferral and Forbearance

This seems like an appropriate place to discuss deferral and forbearance. Along with the federal government, many private lenders offer forbearance and/or deferral (usually just forbearance) in the event of economic hardship. With either option, you do not have to make any payments at all on your student loans. This is obviously great if money is tight. However, remember the difference between the two. With deferral, interest does not accrue on the debt. With forbearance, it does. In other words, the payments you are not making, at least the interest portion, is being added to the loan balance. That "eighth wonder of the world," compound interest, is now working against you. You usually have to apply in some way, but it typically is not difficult for a resident to qualify, at least for forbearance.

Deferral and forbearance are almost never the right move, despite how commonly residents choose these options. Deferral of private loans would not be a bad option, but it is almost never available. The main reason residents tend to put their private loans into forbearance is that they cannot afford the payments until they get an attending-level income. There is now a better solution to this problem. After several years of me bugging them, there are now at least two or three companies that offer a resident student loan refinancing program. In these programs, you are guaranteed a low monthly payment, typically $100, no matter how large your loan is or how high your interest rate is. The rest of the interest due is, of course, tacked on to the loan. But far better to have 5% interest added to the loan than 8% interest. Even a resident can afford $100 a month on their private loans. To see the list of companies currently offering these to residents, visit *The White Coat Investor* recommended student loan refinancing company list mentioned earlier in the chapter.

The bottom line with private student loans is that you should refinance them as soon as you get out of medical school. You will get a few hundred dollars in cash, lower your interest rate, and benefit from payments of $100 per month. As you near residency completion, you can refinance them again to an even lower rate (and get another cash bonus).

FEDERAL STUDENT LOAN MANAGEMENT

Now we turn to a far more complex subject—how to manage your federal student loans. The complexity is a result of the awesome benefits that the federal programs can potentially provide compared to private loans. These benefits include income-driven payments, loan forgiveness, interest subsidies, and protections in the event of death or permanent disability. Sometimes you even get a benefit that you were not expecting, such as the suspension of student loan payments and interest accruals that occurred for nine months in 2020 during the COVID-19 Pandemic. We will tackle each of these benefits in turn.

Income-Driven Repayment Programs

The government recognized that a lot of people had taken out student loans and then ended up with employment situations, whether temporary or long-term, which really did not provide them enough income to pay off those student loans in any sort of reasonable time period. Congress has designed a variety of Income-Driven Repayment (IDR) programs to help with this situation. Only federal student loans qualify for these programs. Any private loans you took out in school or refinanced into are not eligible. With these federal programs, your payments are based only on your income and the number of people in your household. They are not based in any way whatsoever on your total debt nor on your interest rate. Residents routinely enroll in these repayment programs. Frankly, most residents cannot afford to make the "true payments" on their student loans. It is simply impossible to make payments on a 10-year, 7%, $500,000 student loan while earning $50,000 per year. The payments would add up to over $71,000 per year! Even the payments on a 15-year, 5%, $200,000 student loan would total almost $20,000 per year, ⅓ to ½ of a resident's net income.

The first of these IDR programs is called Income-Contingent Repayment, or ICR. This legacy program is almost never used anymore but set the standard for what was to come. Interestingly, this is the only program that does not require you to have a "need" for a lower payment. A borrower of any income is eligible for this program. It also allows Parent PLUS Loans, once consolidated, to be eligible for the program. Under ICR, payments were set at 20% of your "discretionary income." Discretionary income was defined as your adjusted gross income (total income minus above the line deductions like retirement plan contributions) minus 150% of the poverty line (officially the Federal Poverty Guidelines or Level) for your family size and geographic location. For 2020, in the 48 contiguous states, 150% of the poverty line ranged from $19,140 for a single person to $52,740 for a family of six.

Suppose a single resident has an adjusted gross income of $60,000 per year. What would her payments be under the ICR program? $60,000 minus $19,140 = $40,860. $40,860 x 20% = $8,172. If you divide that by twelve months, $8,172/12 = $681 per month. That is still a lot of money for a resident, but it is much less than a regular 10-year payment would be for the typical resident physician. The monthly payment on a 10-year, 7%, $250,000 loan would be almost $3,000 per month. It gets even better if you have a family in residency. Imagine you are married to a stay-at-home spouse and have four children. Now you subtract $52,740 from your $60,000 adjusted gross income, leaving a discretionary income of $7,260. Multiply that by 20% and divide by twelve to get a payment of just $121 per month.

In fact, it is not only possible but common to have IDR payments of $0, particularly that first year when the payment is calculated using your income from the last year of medical school (generally $0). For this reason, many senior medical students file a tax return even though they do not have to, just to be able to "prove" their minimal income for this calculation. Another major benefit of ICR is a forgiveness program. If you make the required payments for 25 years, any debt remaining is forgiven. That sounds great, but there is a catch. The amount forgiven is considered taxable income. If you did not save up the money for this "tax bomb," you may have gone from owing money to the relatively lenient Department of Education to owing money to the relatively demanding Internal Revenue Service.

The second IDR program is called Income-Based Repayment (IBR). While similar to ICR, it came with a major improvement. IBR changed the payments from 20% of discretionary income to 15%. IBR is not used very often anymore, but if a borrower does not qualify for one of the two newer programs, IBR still may be their best option. It is the only option if you have any loans from prior to October 1, 2007, took out no loans after October 1, 2011, or if you have Federal Family Education Loans (FFEL). IBR forgiveness also occurs after 25 years of payments and is fully taxable.

The third IDR program is called Pay As You Earn (PAYE), signed into law in 2012. This program was even more advantageous to borrowers that qualified. The payments dropped to 10% of discretionary income, just half of what they were under the ICR program. In addition, taxable forgiveness came after just 20 years of payments instead of 25. This program is available to current borrowers and anybody that has at least one loan taken out after 2011 and no loans taken out before 2007.

Calculating PAYE and REPAYE Payments					
Household Size	100% of Poverty Line	150% of Poverty Line	Discretionary Income ($60K - 150%)	10% of Discretionary Income	Monthly Payments
1	$12,760	$19,140	$40,860	$4,086	$341
2	$17,240	$25,860	$34,140	$3,414	$285
3	$21,720	$32,580	$27,420	$2,742	$229
4	$26,200	$39,300	$20,700	$2,070	$173
5	$30,680	$46,020	$13,980	$1,398	$117
6	$35,160	$52,740	$7,260	$726	$61

The most recent IDR program is called Revised Pay As You Earn (REPAYE), signed into law in late 2015. This program provides substantial improvements for many borrowers over PAYE, but also several downsides. It preserves the 10% of discretionary income payments. It is also available to all federal loan borrowers, even if they have loans from prior to 2007.

Perhaps its greatest benefit is the potential for a subsidized interest rate. To understand how this works, consider a borrower with a $200,000, 6% student loan. This loan produces approximately $1,000 in interest each month. If the borrower's REPAYE payment were $200, that would leave $800 in unpaid interest. Under ICR, IBR, or PAYE, that $800 would be added to the balance of the loan. Under REPAYE, half of that interest, $400 in this case, is waived, leaving only $400 to be added to the balance of the loan. This subsidy effectively lowers the interest rate of the loan for many borrowers. The higher your loan balance and the lower your payment, the more significant this effect becomes.

Unfortunately, REPAYE comes with three downsides compared to PAYE.

First, the taxable forgiveness aspect of the program is pushed back out to 25 years for graduate and professional school borrowers. While it remains 20 years for undergraduate loans, those loans generally do not represent a very substantial portion of the student loan burden of doctors.

Second, with IBR and PAYE there is a cap on the payments for high earners. If you are in the program and then your income goes up dramatically (as it often does after residency), the payments are capped at the standard 10-year repayment amount. This cap does not exist in the REPAYE program. The higher your income, the higher the payments go.

Third, REPAYE eliminates a strategy some married borrowers use to lower their payments and potentially increase the amount forgiven. These borrowers would file their taxes Married Filing Separately (MFS) rather than Married Filing Jointly (MFJ). While this usually increases the amount of tax paid, it is possible to more than make up for that loss with increased forgiveness.

Due to these downsides, there are still some people for whom PAYE is a better program than REPAYE, complicating student loan management decisions during residency.

Comparison of IDR Programs				
	ICR	**IBR**	**PAYE**	**REPAYE**
Payments	20% of DI*	15% of DI*	10% of DI*	10% of DI*
Eligible for PSLF	Yes	Yes	Yes	Yes
Taxable Forgiveness (undergraduate loans)	25 Years	25 Years (20 for new borrowers)	20 Years	20 Years
Taxable Forgiveness (graduate loans)				25 Years
Must demonstrate need?	No	Yes	Yes	Yes
Parent PLUS eligible?	Yes	No	No	No
FFEL eligible?	No	Yes	No	No

*Discretionary Income (DI)

IDR Forgiveness Programs

While the IDR programs all offer a forgiveness aspect, that forgiveness is not generally very attractive to physician and dentist borrowers. It requires decades of payments before the forgiveness comes and many times the doctors have the student loans paid off before becoming eligible for it. Even if they qualify for it, the forgiveness is taxable as a lump sum in the year it is received, at ordinary income tax rates. Given the typical tax brackets for doctors, the tax bill is not an insignificant sum of money and could be similar in size to the original debt!

Public Service Loan Forgiveness

However, there is a federal student loan forgiveness program that is attractive to many physicians. This program is called Public Service Loan Forgiveness (PSLF). Its requirements are more stringent than the IDR forgiveness programs, but its benefits are also much larger. The forgiveness comes after just 120 monthly payments, or 10 years. It is also tax-free. There is no tax bomb upon receiving it. The remaining debt just goes away.

In order to qualify for PSLF, you must have eligible loans, make 120 on-time payments in a qualifying program, and be employed full-time by a qualifying employer. You must also provide annual certifications from the employer and fill out the PSLF application properly. It is also highly likely that you will have to fight a bit with the federal loan servicing companies in order to receive what you are due. Complying with the requirements of the program over an entire decade, keeping careful records, and ensuring the records of the loan servicing company match yours will require a fair amount of work and hassle. But in the end it may be worth more than the equivalent of an entire year's worth of salary for a physician or dentist. Under current law, there is no cap on the amount forgiven, although there have been proposals in both Congress and presidential budgets to limit this amount.

Eligible loans for PSLF include direct loans, subsidized and unsubsidized Stafford Loans, Parent Loan for Undergraduate Student (PLUS) Loans, and Federal Direct Consolidation Loans. FFEL and Federal Perkins Loans can be eligible if they are consolidated into a Direct Consolidation Loan. Note that PLUS loans can be made to parents or to graduate/professional students themselves. If made to the parent, the rules are slightly different. PSLF eligibility is dependent on the parent's income, not the student's income. They are also not eligible for the IDR programs, except ICR if the loans are consolidated.

Eligible repayment programs for PSLF include all four IDR programs (ICR, IBR, PAYE, and REPAYE), the "10-year Standard Repayment Plan" (note this is different than the 10–30 year long "Standard Repayment Plan for Direct Consolidation Loans"), and in some cases, the Graduated Repayment Plan. In general, if you are going for PSLF your payment plan should be one of the IDR programs, preferably PAYE or REPAYE with their lower payments. If you made 10 years of payments under the 10-year Standard Repayment Plan, there would not be anything left to forgive.

Qualifying employers include non-profit (i.e. 501(c)(3)) and government employers such as the military, public health, the Veterans Administration, Community Health Centers, and similar employers. Note that you must be directly employed, not just an independent contractor with these organizations. Many physicians who work at 501(c)(3) hospitals are actually employed by a for-profit physician group, and would not qualify for PSLF.

Do not forget about the other two requirements: The payments must be made on-time and you must be working full-time. Any late payments or payments made while working part-time do not count toward the 120 payments.

PSLF Requirements
120 monthly payments
On-time payments
Full-time work
Qualifying loans (direct federal)
Qualifying employer (501(c)(3))
Qualifying repayment plan (IDR)

Student Loan Refinancing

Federal student loans can be refinanced to a private lender, usually at a lower interest rate, at any time, including during residency. However, it may not be advisable to do so in some circumstances.

Before we get any further, it is important to understand the difference between consolidation and refinancing. These terms are not interchangeable. If you CONSOLIDATE your federal loans, you are left with a single loan. The interest rates are averaged and then rounded up to the nearest ⅛th of a percentage point. The loans are still eligible for federal programs and federal protections. If you REFINANCE your loans, you generally get a lower interest rate, but the loans are no longer federal loans. They are now private loans, and no longer qualify for IDR programs or forgiveness programs.

In 2020, the Trump administration and Congress ensured that borrowers of federal loans did not have to make payments for a period of nine months (this book is going to press part way through this nine-month period). Those loans also did not accrue interest during this period. Many borrowers who "did the right thing" and refinanced their loans to lower rates prior to this "student loan jubilee" felt misled and betrayed. While this program was obviously helpful to those who still had federal loans (especially those going for PSLF since these nine non-payments count toward their 120 payments), it will leave some borrowers hesitant to refinance because "who knows when the government will do this sort of thing again?" Likewise, you will occasionally hear a politician talk about forgiving all federal student loans. I would caution you against relying on these sorts of unexpected windfalls to manage your student loans. Although nobody knows what the future holds, the likely outcome of staying in federal loan programs when you should otherwise refinance is paying more in interest and being in debt longer.

STUDENT LOAN MANAGEMENT PRINCIPLES

Now that you understand the rules of the various federal programs and the basic principles behind student loan management, it is time to discuss some specific strategies to manage them during residency.

The easiest strategy to understand is to refinance any private student loans as soon as possible. The sooner you refinance them, the sooner the interest rate is lowered and the less you will end up paying on the loans. Just delaying this from the beginning of residency to the end could mean the difference of thousands or even tens of thousands of dollars. While you will still have $100 per month payments that you would not have if you put the loans into forbearance, those payments will be worth it to get a lower interest rate.

Another important principle is to figure out whether or not you will be going for PSLF as soon as possible. While many graduating students are not yet sure if they will work for a qualifying employer, the sooner they can figure this out the easier their student loan planning will become. Trying to keep all options open as long as possible can make for some complicated decision-making. For example, if a resident is not eligible for any significant REPAYE subsidy due to moonlighting or spousal income, it can often make sense to refinance federal student loans during residency.

Many other strategies are designed around maximizing the amount of money forgiven under PSLF. The lower your income, the lower your IDR payments and the more money that will be left to forgive under PSLF. This creates a bit of a perverse incentive. You are now incentivized not to moonlight. You are incentivized not to take the best paying job you can get after residency. Your spouse may be incentivized not to work. You may be incentivized to use a retirement account or health care insurance plan you would not otherwise choose. You may be incentivized to file your taxes in a different way that even results in a higher tax bill. You may also be incentivized to try to avoid grace periods that you might otherwise want to take advantage of. You may be incentivized to take a job you might not otherwise take, or even to complete a fellowship you might not be all that interested in. Since the program takes 10 years, your financial circumstances are likely to change multiple times during that time period, requiring an almost constantly changing strategy to maximize the benefit. It may feel like your entire financial life revolves around PSLF. Especially when combined with the hassle of complying with the demands of the program and fighting the servicing companies to do what they are supposed to do, you can see why some people that would otherwise be eligible for PSLF might just choose to forget about it and just refinance their loans and pay them off themselves instead.

I know that all sounds really complicated, and it can be for certain borrowers. However, these borrowers all have one thing in common—they are married to another person earning a significant amount of income. For convenience sake, let us consider "significant" to be an amount similar to what a resident earns or more. If you are single, or if you are married to a non-earner or a low-earner, student loan management is much simpler. For the most part, you should just refinance your private student loans, enroll in REPAYE for your federal student loans, and put off the decision of whether to go for PSLF until the end of residency when you know what your first job will be.

NINE STUDENT LOAN STRATEGIES YOU SHOULD KNOW

We will now discuss nine specific student loan management strategies that can be used during residency to maximize the amount of money forgiven via PSLF. While some of these only apply to those married to another high earner, most are useful even for a single doctor or one married to a lower earner.

1 – Maximizing the Little Payments

All IDR payments made count toward the 120 required monthly payments, even if those payments are $0 payments. In fact, the more tiny little payments you make, the more you stand to have forgiven in the end. So you definitely do not want to skip or pay late any payments during residency or fellowship. In fact, the longer you spend in training, the more you are likely to have forgiven. You are now being incentivized to do a five-year residency and a couple of one-year fellowships. That will only leave you three (or possibly only two) years of "real payments" to make before the rest is forgiven.

As part of the IDR application process, you have to show what your income is. The easiest way to do this is to use last year's tax return. If you have no income in medical school, but still file a tax return, then as far as the Department of Education is concerned, you have an income of $0 and thus your IDR payments are $0. If you do not have a tax return, you will have to use an Alternative Documentation of Income, usually pay stubs. This will likely result in higher payments for an intern. Thus file a tax return for the prior year during your last few months of school, even if you are not required to.

The IDR reapplication form provides lots of places for you to document that your income went down mid-year, allowing you to lower your payments. However, it does not seem to have any requirement for you to notify the Department of Education that your income went up mid-year. You basically get a pass for the rest of the year every time your income goes up. Thus during your intern year you make payments as if you were a med student, during your PGY2 year you make payments as if you were an intern and so forth. That means that your first year out of residency you are still making payments as if you were a resident. Technically, since the medical year (July to July) is six months off from the tax year (January to December), the year you leave school you pay as a student, the second year you pay as a half-student/half-resident, and finally the third year you pay based on a full resident income.

2 – Skipping the Grace Period

Federal student loans come with a six-month grace period, which surprisingly, is mandatory. You cannot skip it even if you want to. Of course, if you are going for PSLF, you do want to! There is one workaround. That workaround is to consolidate your loans just as soon as you can. As soon as you match in March as an MS4, apply to consolidate your loans. Be sure to specify that you want to consolidate them now, not at the end of the six-month grace period. It will take 4–6 weeks to process, but as soon as it does, you can enroll in your IDR program of choice (usually REPAYE) and start "making" your $0 payments. This technique basically gives you six extra PSLF-qualifying payments. This strategy will be worth different amounts to different people, but with a large loan burden could be worth $20,000 or more in the end.

3 – Contributing to Tax-Deferred Retirement Accounts

In general, somebody in a low tax bracket (at least compared to where they will likely spend their career and even retirement) should preferentially use tax-free (Roth) retirement accounts instead of tax-deferred (traditional) retirement accounts. With a Roth account, you pay the taxes up-front, in a relatively low bracket. With a tax-deferred account, you pay the taxes when you withdraw the money in retirement. While most doctors can withdraw money from tax-deferred accounts at a lower overall tax rate in retirement than they saved when they contributed the money during their peak earnings years, that is not necessarily the case during residency when the doctor has a relatively low income.

However, the federal student loan system has a couple of perverse incentives built into it. For a borrower who is going for PSLF, it can (and generally does) make sense to make tax-deferred contributions during residency. These contributions lower the adjustable gross income that your IDR payments are calculated from. Lower payments mean more debt left to forgive at the end of 10 years. For some people, lower payments can also increase the REPAYE subsidy. That really does not matter for those going for forgiveness (since whatever is left will be forgiven), but it can reduce the total amount paid for someone who does not receive forgiveness.

This technique will likely increase the total tax burden paid, but generally by less than the additional forgiveness amount under most reasonable assumptions. Even for those who do not go for PSLF, the additional REPAYE subsidy will offset the additional taxes and produce a near break-even scenario under most reasonable assumptions.

4 – Filing MFS with PAYE

Another advanced technique used by married borrowers trying to maximize their PSLF is to file taxes Married Filing Separately (MFS) instead of Married Filing Jointly (MFJ). The IRS gives you the choice. While filing MFS usually increases your total tax burden, you are still allowed to select that option. If you are enrolled in PAYE (or IBR for that matter) and file MFS, only your income (rather than your combined household income) is used to calculate your IDR payments. Consider a resident married to an attending. If this couple filed MFJ, their required payment would be quite high, limiting the amount of money left to be forgiven after 10 years of payments. If they filed MFS, at least during residency, the payments will be lower, and the amount of PSLF higher. Like the tax-deferred contribution strategy, this will increase total taxes paid, but perhaps not by as much as it increases the amount forgiven. Remember that under REPAYE, filing taxes MFS does not confer any advantage since the income of both spouses is used to determine the IDR payments.

5 – Refiling Your Taxes

The strategies listed above are generally considered to be ethical methods of managing your student loans by almost everyone. This particular technique, however, falls a bit more into a gray area. The IRS allows you to modify and refile your tax returns for a period of up to three years, using IRS Form 1040X. You are also allowed to recharacterize IRA contributions (traditional to Roth or Roth to traditional) for a period of up to six months after your tax filing date. The US tax system is managed by the Department of the Treasury. The student loan system is managed by the Department of Education. It will probably not surprise you to learn that these two departments do not actually talk to each other. If you prove your income to the Department of Education using your tax forms and subsequently refile your taxes in a way that increases your income but lowers your overall tax burden, nobody at the IRS calls up the Department of Education to let them know. The right hand does not talk to the left.

So some borrowers file their taxes MFS, use those taxes to show their income to the Department of Education, and then later refile their taxes MFJ. Likewise, they may do a traditional IRA contribution and later recharacterize it as a Roth IRA contribution. These moves allow them to have their cake (low IDR payments) and eat it too (low overall tax burden). As near as I can tell, this move is legal and is certainly recommended by multiple student loan specialists. However, it feels unethical and perhaps even fraudulent to me. I would not go this far to maximize my student loan forgiveness.

6 – Using PAYE After Residency

One significant advantage of PAYE over REPAYE is that PAYE has a cap on your IDR payments but REPAYE does not. In some situations, primarily an attending physician or practicing dentist with a relatively low debt-to-income ratio who is going for PSLF, it can be better to be enrolled in PAYE than REPAYE because of this advantage. Particularly if the doctor was not eligible for any significant REPAYE subsidy during training, there is no reason to use REPAYE at all. But for some people, REPAYE will be better for them during training (to get the subsidy) and then PAYE will be better for them after training. Switching from one plan to another is a step that should be planned carefully. Not only does it stop any subsidy you may have been getting, but it will require you to make one "full payment" (i.e. what your payment would be under the 10-year plan) AND it will capitalize any outstanding interest on the loan. While most borrowers have entirely too much fear of capitalizing interest, it would slightly increase the amount one would have to pay back if they were not going for PSLF.

Remember if you are going to change plans, you must change before you become an attending. As an attending with a higher income, you may not qualify for an IDR plan anymore. If you are already in one, you can stay in it, but you cannot enter another one. For this reason, I recommend that if you switch plans you do so before leaving training. Keep in mind this strategy is only right for a very small percentage of doctors. You must

1. Be going for PSLF with all of its requirements and

2. Expect required payments higher than the PAYE cap.

7 – Using a Health Savings Account

Just like contributing to a tax-deferred retirement account can lower your adjusted gross income, so can contributing to a Health Savings Account (HSA). These are some of my favorite investing accounts, since you get a tax-break at the time of contribution, the money grows in a tax-protected way, and then, if you spend it on health care, it comes out of the account tax-free. In order to qualify to use one, you must be using a High Deductible Health Plan (HDHP) and no other health insurance plan. As a general rule, you should select the right health insurance plan first, and then if that plan is an HDHP, use the HSA. However, the fact that using an HSA can also reduce your IDR payments, increase your REPAYE subsidy, and increase the amount of PSLF may sway a few people that otherwise would not use an HDHP/HSA to use one. You simply have to compare the additional forgiveness obtained with the additional cost of healthcare due to higher deductibles. If you already know an HDHP is right for you and are going for PSLF, then do your best to try to max out your HSA each year.

8 – Splitting Your Income in a Community Property State

Arizona, California, Idaho, Louisiana, Nevada, New Mexico, Washington, and Wisconsin are community property states. This generally means that property and income are shared equally between spouses in that state. The rules in every state are a little different, but you generally split your income equally when filing your taxes MFS in these states. So if the higher earner in the couple in one of these states is going for PSLF, they can file MFS and benefit from essentially shifting a bunch of income from the higher earner's tax return to the lower earner's tax return. This reduces the income for the higher earner and thus reduces the required IDR payments, increasing the amount left to be forgiven under PSLF. Keep in mind it does just the opposite for the lower earner. As a clarifying example, if one member of the couple earns $350,000 and the other earns $50,000, they can both file MFS and each claim $200,000 in income. This would decrease the required IDR payment for the higher earner.

9 – PSLF Side Fund

I have saved what I consider to be the most important strategy to the end. There are two significant risks that you undertake when you decide to go for PSLF instead of refinancing your loans and paying them off quickly by living like a resident and dedicating every spare dollar toward the loans.

The first is that you decide you want to do something else for work before you have made the 10 years of payments required for PSLF. Perhaps that something else is working part-time. Remember only payments made while working full-time count toward PSLF. Perhaps that something else is changing to an employer that is not a 501(c)(3) or government employer. Only payments made while employed by a qualifying employer count.

The second risk is what I call legislative risk. This is the risk that the government changes the rules of the game on you. Honestly, I think this risk is fairly low for current borrowers as your promissory notes include the terms of the IDR and PSLF programs. So I think current borrowers will be grandfathered in should any substantial changes to the program take place. This has been the general rule with student loan changes over the years. However, there have been proposals in past presidential budgets to limit PSLF to just $57,000 total and even to eliminate it completely. While it would literally take an Act of Congress to do this, it certainly could happen at some point in the future.

Due to these risks, some doctors who would otherwise qualify for PSLF choose to refinance their loans and pay them back. I think that is the wrong move. A better solution in my opinion is the "PSLF Side Fund." When you have a PSLF Side Fund, you still "Live like a Resident" just like someone paying off their student loans, but you still only pay the minimum on the loans. You take the rest of that money you have carved out of your paycheck and invest it elsewhere. Then, if you choose to change employers or cut back to part-time, or if the government changes the rules and does not grandfather you in, you can simply take that invested money and put it toward your student loans. You will come out a little behind (since you kept your relatively high-rate student loans instead of refinancing), but not too much, especially if you earned a reasonable investing return on that money. If you do get PSLF, that money just becomes part of your retirement savings.

Many people wonder how they should invest their PSLF Side Fund. The safest option is a simple high-interest savings account or a money market fund. If you think there is a high likelihood of using your PSLF Side Fund, I would keep the money safe, even if it earns less. You can also invest the money into bond or even stock index funds. These are still quite liquid and will likely have a higher long-term return. If you think it is unlikely that you will use this money as a PSLF Side Fund, perhaps you want to do that. If you are not otherwise maxing out your retirement accounts, you may even want to use the PSLF Side Fund to do that. Just realize that if you decide to stop going for PSLF, you may want to either carry the debt a little longer or you will have to pay a significant penalty to withdraw from the retirement account. However you invest your PSLF Side Fund, the goal is to build wealth just as quickly no matter whether you went for PSLF and changed your mind or whether you never went for PSLF at all. How that wealth is built (paying down debt or building investments) does not matter as much. Focus on your total net worth rather than the exact composition of that net worth.

Finally, I wanted to include a few brief comments about the IDR forgiveness programs that I recommended against earlier in the chapter. There are a few people, typically those with a very high debt-to-income ratio, who are not willing to take a full-time, PSLF-qualifying job, for whom these programs can work out, even with the massive tax bomb. The key to making it work out is to ensure you are investing enough money on the side to pay that tax bomb. Unfortunately, if you are in such a desperate student loan situation that it makes sense to go for IDR forgiveness, most of your financial life for the next 20–25 years will revolve around obtaining that forgiveness. Seek out professional student loan advice (see link below) if you think this plan could be right for you.

Student loan management in residency is much trickier than it is as a student or as an attending physician or practicing dentist. The rules frequently change and within a few years, some aspects of this chapter may be out of date. Be sure to look up current tax and student loan law and/or seek formal advice before making any high stakes decisions about your loans. If you need help sorting this all out and running the numbers, we keep a list at *The White Coat Investor* of recommended student loan specialists; see the link in the Additional Resources that follow.

MAIN IDEAS

- Private loans can be refinanced at any time thanks to special refinanced loans that allow for $100 payments during residency.

- The default IDR program for most residents should be REPAYE.

- If you are married to another earner and considering PSLF, seek professional advice on managing your student loans.

- If going for PSLF, keep careful records of every payment and every annual employer certification form.

ADDITIONAL RESOURCES

- **Resource:** Cashback Deals on Student Loan Refinancing
  www.whitecoatinvestor.com/student-loan-refinancing

- **Resource:** Student Loan Specific Advisors
  www.whitecoatinvestor.com/student-loan-advice

- **Blog Post:** Ultimate Guide to Student Loan Management for Doctors
  www.whitecoatinvestor.com/ultimate-guide-to-student-loan-debt-management-for-doctors/

- **Blog Post:** Public Service Loan Forgiveness
  www.whitecoatinvestor.com/public-service-loan-forgiveness

- **Blog Post:** REPAYE vs. Refinancing Student Loans as a Resident
  www.whitecoatinvestor.com/repaye-vs-refinancing-student-loans-as-a-resident/

- **Blog Post:** REPAYE vs. PAYE/MFS for Married Residents
  www.whitecoatinvestor.com/repaye-vs-paye-mfs-for-married-residents/

- **Blog Post:** 12 Reasons I Hate IDR Forgiveness Programs
  www.whitecoatinvestor.com/i-hate-income-driven-repayment-forgiveness/

- **Blog Post:** 10 Reasons You Should Pay Off Student Loans Quickly *www.whitecoatinvestor.com/10-reasons-to-pay-off-your-student-loans-quickly/*

- **Blog Post:** PSLF Side Fund *www.whitecoatinvestor.com/pslf-side-fund/*

- **Resource:** Government PSLF Site *studentaid.gov/manage-loans/forgiveness-cancellation/public-service*

- **Resource:** PSLF Application *studentaid.gov/sites/default/files/public-service-application-for-forgiveness.pdf*

- **Resource:** PSLF Employer Certification Form *myfedloan.org/documents/repayment/fd/pslf-ecf.pdf*

CHAPTER SIXTEEN
INVESTING DURING RESIDENCY

Although not as critical to their future financial success as acquiring critical insurance policies, managing student loans properly, and learning to live below their means, residency is also a great time to start investing. Given future earning potential, what a doctor can invest during residency generally will not add up to a large percentage of their future wealth, but it is still important to do for three reasons.

First, you build financial literacy. You can read about investing all day long, but until you actually start investing, there are some aspects you simply will not learn well. For example, you cannot learn your own risk tolerance simply by reading books and discussing investing with others. It really requires the experience of losing real money that you used to own—money that you could have used to buy something you wanted but chose to invest for your future instead. You can learn the basics of retirement accounts and mutual funds and how to use a brokerage account. It is useful to learn this information and develop these skills on relatively small amounts of money. It might seem hard to believe at first, but the skills you use to manage a four-figure portfolio are exactly the same ones you use to manage an eight-figure portfolio.

Second, investing as a resident will build good habits and discipline. Residents often feel like they are poor—like they are living hand to mouth. When you carve money out of your budget, diverting it away from spending and toward the future, you realize that you have more than enough for your needs. In fact, a typical resident salary is the equivalent of the average

American household income. If you cannot invest as a resident, how do you expect most Americans to do so?

Third, a critical aspect of investing is to allow time for compound interest to work. Sometimes referred to as "the eighth wonder of the world," compound interest allows your money to do a substantial portion of the heavy lifting of building your wealth. The money you invest as a resident will have longer to compound than any other dollars you ever invest.

I mentioned above that a resident cannot really get wealthy. That is not entirely true. Imagine a 26-year-old surgery resident that invests $20,000 a year (about ⅓ of her gross income) into tax-free accounts such as Roth 401(k)s or Roth IRAs each year of her five-year residency. If that money earns 8% per year, by the end of residency at age 31, the account will total $117,332. Even if the resident never invests another dollar but continues to earn 8% per year, by 40 the account will be worth $234,547. By 50, that will grow to $506,369. At age 65, the nest egg will be worth over $1.6 million. Turning $100,000 into $1.6 million just by leaving it alone might seem magical, but it demonstrates the benefits of investing early and allowing compound interest to work. Even if you adjust for 3% inflation, the original $100,000 will turn into over $580,000.

Perhaps the best part of investing during residency is that it is the least complicated investing you will ever do. Compared to an attending physician or a dentist in practice for themselves, a resident physician generally has straightforward retirement account options and simple, easy to understand investments available. If ever there was a time you could truly automate your investments, that time is residency. Just set it and forget it!

BEFORE INVESTING

Your best investment as a resident may not be an investment at all. Sometimes part of your salary is tied to your willingness to invest for retirement. This part is often referred to as a "401(k) or 403(b) match." If you put a certain amount of money into the account, your employer will also put a certain amount of money into the account. Failing to get this money is like leaving part of your salary on the table. While every retirement plan is different, a typical match might contribute 50% of the first 6% of your salary that you put into the plan. So if your gross income is $60,000 per year ($5,000 per month), you would need to contribute 6% x $5,000 = $300 per month to the account to get your full match. If you contribute $300, your employer will contribute $150, and at the end of the year you will have $5,400 plus earnings in the account! This money alone may result in your leaving residency with $20,000–$30,000 already invested for retirement.

After receiving your entire salary, there are a few other "non-investments" you should consider. Most residents enter residency with debt they would rather not have. I am not necessarily even talking about student loans here. I am talking about that 8% car loan you took out when your old beater died as an MS3. I am talking about those credit cards you used to fund residency interviews, moving expenses, or that "one last vacation before internship." Outside of getting an employer match, there is no investment that can compare with paying off a 15–30% credit card. Not only does paying off those credit cards pay a high "rate of return," but that rate of return is guaranteed! You do not even have to take any risk to get that return. Most investors would love to have a 15%+ guaranteed investment available to them! Residents often have those and do not even realize it.

Some residents, mostly those who detest debt and know they are not going for student loan forgiveness, do not invest in anything besides paying down their student loans during residency. A 5–8% guaranteed return is nothing to sniff at when money market funds and high yield savings accounts are paying less than 2% a year. If you would prefer to do this, I think that is perfectly reasonable. It is simple, straightforward, and guaranteed. However, it probably will not teach you much about investing, nor allow you to get tax-protected and asset-protected compound interest working for you as soon as possible.

Another important consideration to take before investing is to make sure you are only investing long-term money into long-term investments. The last thing you want to do is to contribute money to your retirement accounts, invest it in the stock market, and then realize you need that money to buy a car or a washing machine. You may end up paying additional tax on that money, pay penalties for the early withdrawal, and perhaps even be forced to sell investments after a decline. Buying high and selling low is not a recipe for investing success. To avoid doing this, make sure you have an emergency fund in place prior to investing anything. Classically, an emergency fund is a liquid, safely invested source of money equal to three to six months of your expenses. If you spend $3,000 per month, $10,000 would be a pretty good emergency fund. This would allow you to fly to your brother's last-minute wedding, purchase a reliable used car, or replace a refrigerator without having to resort to either borrowing or raiding your long-term investing accounts. It might take a while to save up $10,000, and a resident income is awfully stable, but at a minimum I would make sure you have at least enough cash to cover one month of living expenses before investing anything above what is required to obtain any employer match.

You may have other short-term expenses in addition to an emergency fund. For example, many residents (and their partners) look forward to buying a house within six to 12 months of completing training and want to start saving up a down payment toward it during residency. I do not see this as a very high priority for a resident, but if you do, then be sure to invest this money relatively conservatively. Money that you need in less than five years should not be invested in long-term investments like stocks and real estate. Those investments are for long-term goals, like paying for retirement and college for your children. The same principles apply when saving up for a car, a boat, or a dream vacation. Use certificates of deposit (CDs), short-term bond funds, money market funds, or high-yield savings accounts for goals like those.

RETIREMENT INVESTING

Now with these preliminaries out of the way, let us talk about investing long-term money for long-term goals. The main long-term goal you should be thinking about is retirement. Author and former *Wall Street Journal* columnist Jonathan Clements calls this "the greatest challenge of your financial life,"[38] and I agree. A typical physician will wish to have millions of dollars saved up and invested by retirement. I know it seems odd to be thinking about retirement before you have even really started your career, but I assure you that nobody ever regretted starting early on this goal.

I tell attending physicians and practicing dentists that they really need to be saving about 20% of their gross income for retirement in order to preserve their pre-retirement standard of living. If you can do that as a resident, great, but I am far more concerned that residents invest something than exactly how much they invest. If it only works out to be 5–10% of your gross income, that is just fine. Realize that getting that "savings rate" up to 20% will need to be a major financial priority as you move into your career. So really we are talking about saving $3,000–$12,000 per year for a typical resident. If your partner is an ICU nurse or a dentist or an insurance agent, you should be able to do even better. If you have a stay-at-home spouse managing four young children while living in Manhattan, it will probably be less. But for a typical resident, it will be something like $3,000–$12,000 per year.

What type of account should you invest this money into? A retirement account of course! You likely have access to two different types. The first is a 401(k) or 403(b) your employer may offer you. For 2020, you are allowed to contribute $19,500 per year into this account, not including any employer match. It is easy to automate this process. You simply march into the Human Resources office, tell them you want to enroll in the 401(k) plan, and fill out a written or online form telling them to take $500 out of your paycheck every month and put it into the 401(k). It will come off the top of your paycheck so you will not be tempted to spend it. You can then spend or give away the rest of your income guilt-free, knowing you have already "taken care of business."

401(k)s and 403(b)s are named after the section of the tax code that birthed them. In general, you will see 403(b)s offered by non-profit or public employers such as universities and 401(k)s offered by corporations, partnerships, and other for-profit employers. There are slight differences between the two, but they are beyond the scope of this book and rarely matter. Understanding terms like these is part of becoming financially literate. Like medicine, finance has its own language, and until you learn it, it is difficult to even have a conversation with its practitioners. 401(k)/403(b) contributions come in two different flavors, tax-free (Roth) or tax-deferred (traditional). You contribute after-tax dollars into a Roth 401(k) or Roth 403(b). The money then grows tax-free and every dollar taken out of the account in retirement comes out tax-free. Pre-tax dollars are contributed to a traditional 401(k) or traditional 403(b). In this situation, the dollars you contribute are not taxed in the year of the contribution. The account then grows in a tax-protected way and it is not until you withdraw the money in retirement that you pay taxes on it.

If your marginal tax rate at the time of contribution and at the time of withdrawal are equal, it really does not matter which type of contribution you make—you will have the same amount of money after-tax. However, that is rarely the case. Generally, those in a low tax bracket compared to their peak earnings years (i.e. a typical resident) will be better off using a tax-free (Roth) account. Those who are in their peak earnings years (i.e. a typical attending) will be better off using a tax-deferred (traditional) account.

Unfortunately, the federal student loan system has some distorted incentives built into it. The type of retirement account contributions you make can affect your adjusted gross income, and thus the size of your Income-Driven Repayment (IDR) payments. The lower your IDR payments, the higher your REPAYE subsidy may be and the more potential forgiveness you may receive through PSLF or IDR forgiveness plans on those loans. Despite the fact that residents are generally going to be better off tax-wise from using Roth accounts during residency, if they are receiving a substantial REPAYE subsidy or going for PSLF, they are probably still better off making tax-deferred contributions. Note that no matter what type of contribution you make, the employer match is always a tax-deferred contribution.

In addition to any available employer-provided retirement accounts (401(k)s and 403(b)s), you are also allowed to use Individual Retirement Arrangements (IRAs). These accounts have advantages and disadvantages when compared to 401(k)s.

The advantages include lower costs and greater flexibility in the types of investments in the account. You can also contribute to a spousal IRA, even if your spouse does not actually earn any money. In addition, the tax-free (Roth) version of IRAs, unlike 401(k)s, does not require those over 72 to take out Required Minimum Distributions (RMDs).

A major disadvantage of IRAs is a lower contribution limit, in 2021 just $6,000 per person per year for those under 50. While they receive some asset protection benefits from creditors in all states during the bankruptcy process, they often receive less protection than a 401(k). When invested in certain types of leveraged real estate, there can be additional taxes (Unrelated Business Income Tax) due that would not apply in a 401(k). Perhaps most significantly for doctors and other high-income professionals, there are income-based deduction and contribution limits that often ensnare high earners.

For example, if your employer offers you a retirement plan at work, you cannot deduct traditional IRA contributions if you have a modified adjusted gross income (MAGI) over $76,000 ($125,000 MFJ, $10,000 MFS) in 2021. Even if just your spouse has a plan available at work, you cannot deduct your contribution if your MAGI is over $208,000. On the Roth IRA side, a 2021 MAGI of greater than $140,000 ($208,000 MFJ, $10,000 MFS) prevents you from contributing directly to a Roth IRA. A workaround that many doctors use is called a Backdoor Roth IRA, which consists of contributing to a traditional IRA (no deduction) and then converting it to a Roth IRA later (at no tax cost). However, this indirect Roth IRA contribution process is subject to a pro-rata rule that requires you to roll traditional and SEP-IRAs into a 401(k) or similar plan. These downsides are certainly hassles associated with IRAs.

So what is a resident investor to do about all of these retirement accounts? Well, the solution is typically pretty easy. Most residents do not earn and save enough to max out both a 401(k) ($19,500 employee contribution for 2021) and an IRA ($6,000 for 2021). Their entire annual investment may fit into either account with room to spare. Obviously, if your employer offers a match you want to contribute enough to the employer plan to get the entire match. After that, it is fine to use an IRA for your next $6,000 of retirement savings each year. If you are receiving a significant REPAYE subsidy or going for PSLF, use the tax-deferred (traditional) version of these plans. If you are not, use the tax-free (Roth) version.

Just be aware when using IRAs that if your MAGI is too high that you might as well use a Roth IRA since you cannot deduct a traditional IRA contribution anyway. Things change a bit when you become an attending. You will definitely want to save more money; I recommend attendings put at least 20% of their gross income toward retirement. You will also need to start funding your Roth IRAs "through the backdoor." Due to the pro-rata rule, you will eventually need to do something with any traditional IRA that you have at that time. Your options are usually to either roll it over into a future 401(k) or pay the taxes and convert it all to a Roth IRA. More information about the Backdoor Roth IRA process can be found at *www.whitecoatinvestor.com/backdoor-roth-ira-tutorial/*.

THE THREE CATEGORIES OF INVESTMENTS

Now that we have sorted out where you should invest, we should talk about what to invest in. Many doctors have trouble understanding the difference between investment accounts and investments. A 401(k) and a Roth IRA are investment accounts. Stocks, bonds, mutual funds, and real estate are investments. Think of an investment account as luggage and investments as clothes. Generally, any investment can go into any type of investment account, just like any piece of clothing can go into any piece of luggage. Obviously, some types of luggage and some types of clothing are more appropriate for different types of trips, so it is important to learn the advantages and disadvantages of each type and use them properly.

There are generally three types of investments:

1. Productive Assets
2. Interest-Paying Instruments
3. Speculative Instruments

Productive assets include the ownership of companies that provide goods and services, including real estate companies that provide a place for people to live or businesses to operate. These companies can be owned in whole or in part. When publicly-traded, partial ownership (shares) of these companies are often called "stocks." You can buy and sell these shares on the stock market any day the market is open. Ownership is considered a relatively risky form of investment. If the company does well, you get to share in the profits. They often come in the form of dividends or rents. If the company does poorly, you get to share in the losses, including the potential loss of your entire investment. About 26,000 companies in the US go bankrupt each year. Even large, profitable, publicly-traded companies go bankrupt each year—58 in 2018, and 64 in 2019, a year when the overall stock market provided nearly 30% returns![39]

Interest-paying instruments include savings accounts, certificates of deposit, money market funds, bonds, and similar investments. Rather than ownership, these investments are loans to an individual, company, or government. While some are riskier than others, interest-paying instruments are generally considered to be less risky than productive assets. You are less likely to lose your investment, but you are also likely to earn a lower rate of return over the long run.

Speculative instruments are anything you buy that does not have any sort of earnings or pay any interest. Purchasers of these investments (and I am hesitant to even call most of them investments at all) hope to later sell the instrument to someone else for a higher price than they paid for it. These investments include non-productive land, currencies (Euros, Yen, etc.), cryptocurrencies (Bitcoin, Ethereum, Ripple), precious metals (gold, silver), Beanie Babies, baseball cards, art, and other collectibles.

As a general rule, the long-term investments of a resident should be primarily composed of productive assets. The consequences of loss on your relatively tiny portfolio are minimal, and the amount of time to recover any temporary losses is as long as it ever will be. As you move throughout your career and approach financial independence, you may wish to gradually add interest-paying instruments to the mix. It will reduce the volatility of the portfolio and provide diversification. These safer investments tend to zig when productive assets like stocks or real estate zag in a market downturn. Speculative instruments should generally be avoided. If you cannot help yourself, at least limit these to a single-digit percentage of your portfolio.

THE CASE FOR MUTUAL FUNDS

One of the easiest, safest, and most convenient ways to invest in any of these types of investments is using mutual funds. A mutual fund is essentially a group of investors that pools their money together to invest. This pooling allows them to benefit from economies of scale, hire professional management, provide easy diversification, and enjoy convenient liquidity. Mutual funds are an ideal way to invest, both for beginners and sophisticated investors. The vast majority of serious investors use mutual funds for their serious money. In fact, many employer-provided retirement plans do not offer individual investments like stocks and bonds; they only offer mutual funds.

There are two general types of mutual funds, actively-managed and passively-managed. In an actively-managed stock fund, the manager tries to buy the best stocks and avoid the worst stocks. Using a highly-talented staff of analysts and high-powered computer programs, the goal is to achieve higher returns at lower levels of risk. A passively-managed stock fund takes a different approach. Rather than trying to beat the market averages, this type of fund simply tries to match the market return. This is relatively easy and inexpensive to achieve. Since the market is composed primarily of talented active managers competing against each other to outperform the market, it turns out that it is now quite difficult to outperform the market over the long-term, especially once you consider the costs (including taxes) of doing so. The data is quite clear that over the long run you are much more likely to have higher investment returns with passive funds than active funds.[40] Passive funds are also frequently called index funds, and savvy investors primarily use these in their portfolios. Index funds are inexpensive, avoid certain types of risks such as manager risk, outperform most active funds investing in the same asset class over the long run, and are very tax-efficient.

A SIMPLE, SOPHISTICATED SOLUTION

Residents are busy folks, often have little education or understanding of finance and investing, and have all of their investments inside one or two tax-protected investment accounts. An ideal investment for an investor like this is referred to as a fund of funds, balanced fund, lifecycle fund, or target date fund. These mutual funds are basically a single mutual fund that buys a handful of other mutual funds to provide easy diversification and automatic rebalancing. They are a surprisingly sophisticated one-stop shop for the new investor. Investor-owned mutual fund powerhouse Vanguard offers two of my favorite types of these—Target Retirement funds (which become less aggressive as you age) and Life Strategy funds (which maintain the same mix of investments over time). Either of these makes for an excellent first investment. You will own every publicly traded stock and bond in the world with a single purchase. If you open an IRA or Roth IRA at Vanguard, these will be easy choices for you and then you can get back to your important clinical training. Your employer 401(k)/403(b) likely offers similar investments. While I built my own portfolio of index funds during residency, if I had it all to do over again, I would have just kept it ultra-simple and used one of these funds, at least until my training was complete.

Many doctors, including some busy residents, become interested in real estate investing. While you can invest in publicly-traded real estate using index mutual funds, you do miss out on some of the control and tax benefits of investing directly. Unfortunately, investing directly is the equivalent of running your own company, which requires both time and expertise to do well. Few residents have much of either to spare. Land lording has many aspects of a second job, and most residents are already working the equivalent of two full-time jobs. If you are interested in real estate investing, I would encourage you to concentrate on your clinical training for now and leave it for your attending years. There will be plenty of time (and far more money) you can use to become a real estate magnate later, I promise.

The most important aspect of investing for residents is simply to get into the habit and cultivate a consistent practice. If you will invest something every month as a resident, you are likely to carry that habit forward into your attending years. Almost every investor wishes they had started earlier because time in the market beats trying to time the market, and the only way to maximize your time in the market is to get that money into the market as soon as possible.

While investing should not be a major focus for residents, learning the language and getting started early will provide life-long benefits. Take advantage of the tax-protected and asset-protected accounts available to you and choose low-cost, broadly-diversified, automatic, passive mutual fund investments that allow you to build wealth relatively safely with little effort.

MAIN IDEAS

- Starting to save and invest for retirement in residency builds excellent habits for the future.

- The earlier you start investing, the longer compound interest has to work.

- If your employer offers a 401(k) or 403(b) match, be sure to contribute enough to their retirement plan to receive the whole match.

- Invest in Roth accounts (IRA, 401(k), 403(b) preferentially as a trainee) unless going for PSLF or receiving a large REPAYE subsidy.

- Sometimes your best investment is paying off debt or saving up an emergency fund to prevent you from going back into debt.

- A simple investing plan can be very sophisticated and easy to manage.

ADDITIONAL RESOURCES

- **Blog Post:** Pay Off Debt or Invest
  www.whitecoatinvestor.com/pay-off-debt-or-invest/

- **Blog Post:** Financial Lessons for Residents by a Resident
  www.whitecoatinvestor.com/financial-lessons-for-residents/

- **Blog Post:** Yes, Residents Can Save for Retirement
  www.whitecoatinvestor.com/yes-residents-can-save-for-retirement/

- **Blog Post:** Why Everyone Should Love the Roth IRA
  www.whitecoatinvestor.com/why-i-love-the-roth-ira-back-to-basics/

- **Blog Post:** Roth vs. Traditional When Going for PSLF
  www.whitecoatinvestor.com/roth-vs-traditional-pslf/

CHAPTER SEVENTEEN

PROTECTING YOUR MOST VALUABLE ASSET

A practicing dentist or physician has the potential to earn $200,000–$500,000 per year for the next 30–40 years. This represents a sum of $6–$20 million. Converting this potential income and wealth into actual income and wealth is the greatest financial task of your life. However, there are risks that could show up in your life that would prevent you from being able to accomplish this task. One of the most common of these risks is an extended or even permanent disability. Insurance companies estimate that as many as one in seven doctors will be disabled at some point during her career. While many imagine this will occur in a sudden traumatic accident, medical illness is actually a more common cause of disability that prevents a doctor from working.

Some disabilities are only partial disabilities, where the doctor is still able to either work part-time or is only able to perform some of the duties of their occupation. Disabilities can last just a few weeks or can be lifelong. Most doctors do not have the skills or education to generate anywhere near their former income doing anything besides the practice of medicine or dentistry. They invested 10–15 years in their education and training to develop their specialized knowledge base and skill set. Not insuring this ability against such a prevalent risk with such serious consequences is simply foolish.

Disability insurance protects you and your loved ones in the event that a disability prevents you from working. If you become disabled, a long-term disability insurance policy pays a predetermined amount each month until you either recover from your disability or reach age 65–67 (policies vary).

Insurance companies limit the amount of your income that you can insure, typically to approximately 60% of your prior gross income. However, since the insurance benefit is generally tax-free and working doctors are typically paying 20–30% of their income in taxes, most insured doctors can still have a very nice life living on their disability benefits. While insurance companies might like to sell you an even larger policy, they also do not want to make going on disability too attractive, thus the 60% limit.

Since disability insurance is frequently used, it tends to carry fairly expensive premiums. Typically, a solid policy will cost you 2–6% of the benefit. So if you purchase a policy with a $10,000 per month benefit, expect to pay $200–$600 per month. This will be a major budget line item for you during your career, so try to get over the sticker shock quickly. Many doctors justify purchasing less insurance, purchasing less comprehensive insurance, or not purchasing disability insurance at all because performing procedures does not generate a significant portion of their practice. This is a mistake since this factor is already "baked in" to the pricing of a policy; proceduralists (including dentists) pay more for their policies. Good policies are own-occupation, specialty-specific policies. This means that they will pay you the promised benefit in the event that you cannot perform the essential duties of your specialty, even if you could do something else. Each specialty is placed into its own risk category. Surgeons and dentists tend to fall into the riskier, more expensive categories. Psychiatrists and preventive medicine docs tend to fall into the least risky, least expensive categories.

OWN-OCCUPATION, SPECIALTY-SPECIFIC

The most important aspect of a policy is the definition of disability. Life insurance, which pays out a lump sum to your beneficiary if you die, is very simple in comparison to disability insurance. Determining if someone is alive or dead is relatively easy. By comparison, disability involves many shades of gray. Determining if someone is too disabled to perform their job can be complicated. As a result, disability insurance contracts tend to be complicated. As discussed above, the strongest definition of disability is "own-occupation." However, there are other definitions available including "modified own-occupation," "medical own-occupation," and "any occupation." An example of any occupation is Social Security Disability Insurance (SSDI). If you can work at any job, it will not pay. Despite large numbers of people in our society being on SSDI, it is surprisingly difficult to qualify for because you can be quite disabled and still be able to do something.

Medical own-occupation is a definition used by just one company (whose policies I do not recommend), which bases your benefits on the amount of income lost rather than the loss of the ability to do the essential duties of your occupation. In reality, it is simply another version of modified own-occupation, which will pay you if you cannot perform the essential duties of your occupation AND you do not work at any other occupation. The stronger the definition of disability, the more expensive the policy, but also the more likely it is to actually pay you in the event of disability. I see little reason for a doctor to pay a lot of money for a policy that does not have the best definition of disability available—own-occupation, specialty-specific.

There are six companies currently selling true own-occupation policies to doctors including Principal, The Standard, Guardian, Ameritas, Mass Mutual, and Ohio National. The good news is that you do not have to meet with an agent from each of these companies to compare. You can simply select a broker (also known as an independent agent) who can sell you a policy from any of these companies and help you compare one to another. You can find a list of recommended agents here:

Resource: Recommended Insurance Agents
www.whitecoatinvestor.com/insurance

There are two main types of disability policies: individual policies and group policies. As a general rule, individual policies have stronger definitions of disability. Many group policies are not own-occupation policies. Individual policies are also portable, in that you can change jobs and take them with you. A group policy provided by your employer is usually not portable, although sometimes you are allowed to take over the entire premium and take it with you. Group policies also frequently have premiums that increase every year or every five years, whereas an individual policy usually has level premiums. Group policies paid for by your employer may also pay a taxable benefit, rather than the tax-free benefit provided by an individual policy. Aside from lower cost, the only benefit of a group policy is that it may be easier to qualify for. It may not require any sort of medical exam or blood work, and may not ask any pesky questions about your medical conditions and dangerous hobbies such as rock climbing, skydiving, SCUBA diving, or flying.

WHEN TO BUY DISABILITY INSURANCE

Medical students actually can buy disability insurance (and some schools even provide it). However, in my opinion, the time to purchase it is when you first start earning money, i.e. as an intern. I am absolutely appalled to run into senior residents, young attendings, and even mid-career attendings who need disability insurance but have not actually purchased any. For this reason, the first chapter in my last book (*The White Coat Investor's Financial Boot Camp*) was all about disability insurance. It is that important.

As you leave medical school and move into residency, this is your greatest financial priority. Residents get disabled all the time and even though you may only qualify to purchase (or be able to afford) a $5,000 benefit, that benefit will be a lifesaver if you become disabled. If it is already past your first Halloween in residency and you do not have disability insurance, you have dropped the ball. Get it done. If you need help, we maintain a list of recommended independent insurance agents at *www.whitecoatinvestor.com/insurance*. These agents sell hundreds of policies a year to white coat investors just like you. They will help you find the best policy for your unique situation.

Another great reason to buy a disability insurance policy now is that it will probably never be as cheap for you as it is today. The price goes up as you get older and acquire medical conditions. Pricing does vary by state (for example California is a particularly bad state in which to buy insurance), gender (policies for men are cheaper than policies for women so women should look for a gender-neutral policy, although companies seem to be phasing these out), medical condition (although most are simply excluded from the policy rather than priced in), and dangerous hobbies (also usually simply excluded from coverage).

RIDERS

Most policies also include some riders. Think of a rider as an additional benefit that you can purchase for an additional premium once you have purchased the base policy. Every purchaser should buy a partial/residual disability rider. This provides a partial benefit to you in the event of a partial disability or during the recovery from a complete disability. Resident purchasers will also want to buy two other riders. The first is a cost of living rider. This rider increases the benefit each year with inflation beginning with the year after you are disabled. The second rider is a future purchase option rider. This allows you to buy a larger policy when your income goes up (usually when you become an attending) without a medical questionnaire or exam. This is important in case you do develop a medical problem during your training. If you are still healthy, you can simply buy a second policy. But if you are not, your only option for additional coverage will be exercising that rider. You can always drop the rider in a few years if you want to save that additional premium. These policies usually offer other riders including student loan riders, retirement riders, and catastrophic disability riders. I generally recommend against these for most doctors, but you can discuss their advantages and costs with your agent and make the decision for yourself.

Recommended Disability Insurance Riders	
Rider	Recommendation
Partial/Residual Disability	Yes for all
Future Purchase Option	Yes for residents
Cost of Living Adjustment	Yes if under 50 years old
Student Loan	No (buy a larger base benefit instead)
Retirement	No (buy a larger base benefit instead)
Catastrophic	No (buy a larger base benefit instead)

Most purchasers of a disability insurance policy will qualify for some type of discount. Most commonly it is a group discount available to every doctor at your training hospital. Be sure to ask for one. If your agent does not offer one, it may be worth getting a second opinion from another agent. Aside from those discounts, there is little reason to use multiple independent agents as the base policies are all priced the same.

Remember that there are lots of ways to lose your ability to practice medicine; disability is just one of them. Neither your disability nor your malpractice insurance will help you if you lose your ability to practice due to losing your license, losing your board certification, losing your hospital credentials, insurance or Medicare fraud, criminal acts, or sexual harassment.

Nevertheless, disability is common enough among physicians that you should carry a policy from the time you leave school until the time you reach financial independence.

MAIN IDEAS

- Your most valuable asset is your ability to trade your time for money at a very high rate for the next few decades. Insure it as soon as you come out of school.

- The best policy is an individual, portable, own-occupation, specialty-specific policy.

- Purchase disability insurance from an independent agent who can show you policies from all of the major companies.

- Buy as much disability insurance as they are willing to sell you as a resident. Include a future purchase option and a cost of living rider. You will probably buy more when you finish training.

ADDITIONAL RESOURCES

- **Resource:** Recommended Independent Insurance Agents
  www.whitecoatinvestor.com/insurance

- **Blog Post:** What You Need to Know About Physician Disability Insurance
  www.whitecoatinvestor.com/what-you-need-to-know-about-disability-insurance/

- **Blog Post:** 17 Physician Disability Insurance Mistakes
  www.whitecoatinvestor.com/physician-disability-insurance-mistakes/

- **Blog Post:** Disability Insurance for Military Physicians
  www.whitecoatinvestor.com/disability-insurance-for-military-physicians/

- **Blog Post:** Disability Insurance for Two Doctor Couples
  www.whitecoatinvestor.com/disability-insurance-for-two-doctor-couples/

CHAPTER EIGHTEEN

GOT DEPENDENTS?
GET LIFE INSURANCE

Many people are married and/or have children by the time they are done with their medical or dental training. Partners often make significant sacrifices in order to support you in pursuing your dream. These sacrifices may be personal and difficult to quantify, but are often easily-quantified financial and career-related sacrifices. Just like you, they invested this time and money into your future earning ability. Their investment should be protected, particularly if they are dependent on your future income to maintain their standard of living. This especially applies to your children. While people do not die young very often (about 1% of people die in their 30s), that number is not zero.

While you can never be replaced in the event of an untimely death, your income can. The financial instrument that does this is called life insurance. If someone else depends on your income, you need to buy some life insurance. Pure, or "term," life insurance is a very simple product. You pay a premium every month or year and if you die during that month or year, a death benefit is paid out to your beneficiary. The beneficiary can then use this money to pay off a mortgage, send a child to college, start a career or business, or simply to invest for future living expenses.

Some term insurance policies are annually renewable, meaning the price goes up each year, while others are level premium, meaning the premium remains the same for a period of time ranging from 5–30 years. Most level premium policies can be extended beyond the 30-year period, but then become an annually renewable policy. The jump in price from year 30 to year 31 is usually pretty dramatic, however, so it is best to make sure you buy a policy with a long enough term that you are certain you will be financially independent by the time the term is up. Once you have a nest egg sufficient to support your loved ones in the event of your death, you have no need for life insurance and can safely cancel the policy and save the premium.

Most people are dramatically underinsured because they have no understanding of just how much money is needed to live for decades without earning money. If your goal is for your spouse to never work again, consider how much your spouse will need to spend per year after your death and multiply by 25. If you have substantial savings, you can subtract that amount at this point. You may also wish to add an additional amount such as enough to pay off a mortgage or pay for a college education for children. Most residents who do this calculation will arrive at a seven-figure number. At that point, round up to the next million, just to be safe.

Doctors with dependents likely have a life insurance need somewhere between $1 million and $5 million. The good news is that even that much insurance is relatively cheap to a young, healthy resident. A 26-year-old healthy female can buy $1 million of 30-year level premium term life insurance for just $460 per year, or about $40 per month. This is dramatically cheaper than disability insurance and there is little excuse to not buy at least a $1 million policy as a resident if anyone else is depending on you.

Typically, a term life policy is purchased from the same independent agent who sold you your disability insurance policy. The application, medical/ hobby questions, and medical exam are very similar. One difference between the policies is what happens with medical issues or dangerous hobbies. A disability policy generally excludes these conditions from coverage, meaning if you become disabled rock climbing and have a rock-climbing exclusion, the policy will not pay. A life policy does not exclude conditions, it simply charges you more for the policy (or does not issue it to you at all). With either policy, you do not want to be formally turned down for insurance. An experienced agent will shop you around to companies informally to prevent you from having a denial on your record, and then formally apply only when it looks very likely that you will be approved. You are not only required to disclose denials when you apply for insurance in the future, but the industry keeps a database with any denials issued by any company.

Besides term life insurance, there are also various kinds of permanent or "cash value" life insurance. The best known of these is whole life insurance, but there are other types including universal life, variable life, variable universal life, and index universal life insurances. Each of these policies has a life-long death benefit, meaning it will pay your beneficiaries even if you die at age 95. As you might imagine, insuring people who are actually likely to die costs a lot of money, and so the premiums for these permanent policies are often 10–20 times as expensive as a term policy. The biggest problem thus becomes that people who mistakenly buy permanent insurance instead of term insurance end up being underinsured. They simply cannot afford all of the insurance they need at the price charged for a permanent life insurance product.

So why do companies and agents sell permanent life insurance, especially when so few people actually have a need for a permanent death benefit? Well, it turns out it is very profitable to do so. A permanent policy is much more expensive and thus the agent commissions are much higher. A typical insurance agent commission on a whole life insurance policy ranges from 50–110% of the first year's premium. So if an agent can talk a doctor into purchasing a policy with a $30,000 annual premium, that agent could be paid as much as $30,000 for doing so!

These agents use many different sales tactics to sell these policies. While beyond the scope of this book, you can learn more in a series of blog posts found here:

Blog Post: Debunking the Myths of Whole Life Insurance
www.whitecoatinvestor.com/debunking-the-myths-of-whole-life-insurance/

Most of the sales points involve borrowing against the death benefit in order to do something else with the money. The bottom line is that very few doctors need a whole life insurance policy and most of them do not want one once they actually understand how they work. I view selling a whole life insurance policy to a resident (or worse, a student like I was when one was sold to me) as the equivalent of malpractice for insurance agents.

Buying life insurance if you have dependents is part of being a financially responsible adult. If you have dependents, this needs to be a major priority at the beginning of your first year of residency. Get a $1–$5 million, 30-year level term policy in place as soon as possible.

MAIN IDEAS

- If anyone else depends on your income besides you, buy term life insurance to protect them.

- Few doctors need or want a whole life insurance policy, and no student or resident needs one.

- Term life insurance purchased when you are young and healthy is very inexpensive. Buy at least $1 million in coverage.

ADDITIONAL RESOURCES

- **Resource:** Recommended Independent Insurance Agents
  www.whitecoatinvestor.com/insurance

- **Blog Post:** How to Buy Life Insurance
  www.whitecoatinvestor.com/how-to-buy-life-insurance/

- **Blog Post:** Term Life Insurance Strategies for Physicians
  www.whitecoatinvestor.com/term-life-insurance-strategies-for-physicians/

- **Blog Post:** Term Life Insurance: What You Need to Know Before You Buy
  www.whitecoatinvestor.com/term-life-insurance-what-you-need-to-know-before-you-buy/

- **Blog Post:** What You Need to Know About Whole Life Insurance
  www.whitecoatinvestor.com/what-you-need-to-know-about-whole-life-insurance/

PART THREE

THE NEXT STEP: ACHIEVING FINANCIAL LITERACY

In this third section of the book, I am going to provide you a crash course of high-yield information that you will eventually want to know. Unlike the first two sections of the book, which contain specific pieces of advice and recommendations, this section is composed primarily of background information that will allow you to better understand and implement those recommendations.

Most financial books spend their first 100–200 pages teaching you the basics of personal finance and investing, and then in the last chapter or two actually tell you what to do with your money. This is so frequently true that you can usually just read the last few chapters of a book to really understand an author's take, since the first ¾ of the book is the same as most other books you will find. I decided to turn that philosophy on its head. In the first section of the book, I told you everything you need to know during medical or dental school and what to do with your finances during those four years. In the second section of the book, I gave you a look ahead to residency, especially the beginning of residency, and listed out the critical financial tasks that will ensure your financial security if you will complete them. In this last section of the book, I want to take you on a journey toward financial literacy.

Financial literacy is not only very rare, but also incredibly valuable. Once you understand how the financial world works, it may feel like you have a superpower. You will look at the world around you and wonder why the people surrounding you seem to be continually making terrible financial decisions. A big part of it is that they simply do not know what you will soon know. A little knowledge goes a long way, and in the remainder of the book I am going to provide a high-yield, no-nonsense guide to maximize the bang for your buck.

In my opinion, there are three important aspects of financial literacy. The first involves learning the language of finance. If you cannot speak finance, it is difficult to even have a conversation with another investor or advisor. The first two chapters in this section, the first on investments and the second on investment accounts, will help you learn that language.

The second aspect of financial literacy and the third chapter in this section is knowing a bit about the history of financial markets. History might not repeat, but it certainly rhymes.[51] History informs you as to the range of possible outcomes you might see over your investing career and prepares you to weather the inevitable economic downturns. It turns out that investing success depends a lot more on the investor than it does on the investment, and knowing history makes you a more rational, more patient, and more successful investor.

The third aspect of financial literacy and the fourth chapter in this section involves a bit of math. Luckily, you learned most of the math you need to be a successful investor in elementary school. No algebra, geometry, or calculus required here. If it involves more than simple addition, subtraction, multiplication, division, and percentages, you can simply use a financial calculator.

If you enjoy learning this information, remember there is more of it available than you will find here. This section is the "100 level" (101, 102, 103, 104) financial literacy material. If you find it useful, I will send you the "200 level" (201, 202, 203, 204) courses absolutely free. Sign up at *www.whitecoatinvestor.com/bonus*.

SIGN UP NOW

CHAPTER NINETEEN

STOCK, BONDS, AND MUTUAL FUNDS

(FINANCIAL LITERACY 101)

I wish there were a way to make this subject incredibly exciting. I have read dozens of investing books over the years, and I still do not think I have ever seen anyone make this subject as exciting as a good novel, much less a blockbuster movie. Nobody binge-watches "stocks and bonds." However, I did not particularly find Physics or Histology exciting either, but I still learned them because I knew I had to in order to do what I wanted to do with my life.

So I am going to bribe you to read this material. No, I am not going to send you a check if you manage to make it through these financial literacy chapters. I am going to pay you with your own money. When combined with a physician or dentist income over a career, a working knowledge of the basics of investing is likely worth a couple of million dollars. Even if it takes you four hours to get through the rest of this book, that is still an hourly rate of $500,000 per hour. Think about that minimum wage job you used to have and all the hours you poured into it. Now, are you sure you are not willing to put four hours into this book if you are paid $500,000 per hour to read it? I thought that might provide the motivation you needed.

In an earlier chapter of this book we briefly discussed three types of investments—productive assets, interest-bearing instruments, and speculative instruments. This overall framework is helpful when learning more about individual investments. You can also place these types of investments onto a spectrum of risk, from least risky to most risky. Note that while the general rule is that more risk usually equals a higher expected return, that is not always true, particularly as you get into speculative instruments. Sometimes taking on higher risk does not usually lead to a higher return. You have to be smart about the risks you take.

The Investment Risk Spectrum

Savings Account
Certificate of Deposit (CDs)
Money Market Fund
Short Term Treasury Bonds
Long Term Treasury Bonds
Unleveraged Real Estate
Stocks
Small Cap Value/ Emerging Market Stocks
Leveraged Real Estate
Precious Metals
Cryptocurrency

LOW RISK

HIGH RISK

PRODUCTIVE ASSETS

Perhaps the most common type of productive asset owned by investors is a publicly traded stock. Remember when you own a share of stock, you are a partial owner of a company. Your financial fortunes are now tied to those of the company. If Apple, General Electric, or Exxon does well, the investors do well. The investors are the company.

Modern politicians and activists love to malign the "evil corporations" who are taking all of our money. In reality, the "evil corporations" are you and me. The evil corporations are your child's teacher's pension, your retirement account, and your niece's college fund. Thus, any tax on a corporation is really a tax on the people who own it. It simply shows up in the form of lower returns. All taxes are personal in the end. Obviously, a tax on a corporation is going to fall most heavily on those who own corporations. The wealthier you are, the larger the percentage of the world's corporations that you own. So in that sense, a corporate tax is simply another progressive tax that falls most heavily on the wealthy.

I often encourage people to think and act "like an owner." The more you act like an owner, the sooner you are likely to be an owner. Employees who think like an owner care about the customers, the equipment, fellow employees, and the success of the company. In short, they treat the company like it is their own. People with ownership mentality take smart, calculated risks and go the extra mile. They come early, stay late, and rejoice in maximizing the success of the enterprise. When an owner finds an employee who really cares about the business, the employee is promoted and promoted again. They eventually learn the entire business. They may be offered equity in the business or may leave the company to open a competing business. They know that when the business is successful, the lion's share of the benefits flow to the owners. They extend this knowledge to their investments.

The sooner you start thinking like an owner, the sooner you can benefit from owning pieces of the most profitable corporations the world has ever seen. For example, in 2019 Microsoft earned $39 billion in profit.[41] That is more money than the Gross Domestic Product (GDP) of half of the countries in the world.[42] It is about the same as the GDP of all of Wyoming.[43] A large part of the increased standard of living we enjoy compared to those who lived 300–400 years ago is a result of the work of corporations. Now you too can own (an admittedly tiny) piece of these corporations.

VALUING COMPANIES

Imagine you started a business. If you make smart decisions, work hard, and have a little luck, your business may become successful and start making money. Perhaps the business made $200,000 in a year. It was fun to earn that reward and it was fun to be able to provide a living for your employees and to support other partnering businesses. But now you would like to do something else. You want to move on with your life, but you own this business. How can you do that? Well, first you must replace yourself. Perhaps you can hire a manager to run your business for $100,000 a year. Now you are free of the business and it still provides you a relatively passive income of $100,000 per year. A business that spits off $100,000 a year without any effort from you is a beautiful and valuable thing. But how valuable is it?

Well, that depends on a lot of things. It depends on whether that $100,000 in profit is likely to go up or go down. It depends on the stability of the revenue and expenses. If all of your profit came from a single event that is unlikely to be repeated, then it is not as valuable. If your factory needs to be completely renovated, it is not as valuable. But in general, most profitable businesses can be valued as a multiple of their profit (or earnings). A small, risky, insecure business might be valued at a multiple of five times its profit. That might be appropriate for this small business of yours. If it earns $100,000 per year, the company would be worth $500,000. A larger, more stable company might be valued at 20 times its earnings. If it earned $1 billion a year, it would be worth $20 billion.

This type of calculation is inherent in valuing any company and you can calculate this number for any publicly traded stock in the world. It is called the Price to Earnings ratio, or P/E ratio. The better the prospects of a company, the higher that P/E ratio ought to be. A company with excellent products, little competition, and prospects for rapid growth might have a P/E ratio of 30, 50, or even 100. In the stock market, these companies are called "growth stocks." A company without the same advantages, even if profitable, may have a P/E ratio of just 8–10. These are called "value stocks." One might intuitively think that it would be smart to own growth stocks instead of value stocks. Surely your return will be better if you just buy the high flyers. However, the truth is that an investor should be agnostic toward the type of investment owned. At the right price, a slow-growing company is just as good of an investment as a fast-growing company. If the P/E ratio is right for the company, you will do just as well owning value stocks as growth stocks. Thus the key lies in properly valuing the company.

How much should an investor pay for a dollar of that company's earnings? This is the question millions of investors are asking themselves every day when buying and selling stocks. Is this company worth a P/E ratio of 15 or of 20? The price for a share of the company is determined by the consensus decision of all of those investors about this question. It is the price at which half of them are willing to sell and half of them are willing to buy. Bad news for the company or even the overall economy will cause that price to fall. Good news will cause it to rise. But that price is determined by the market, i.e. the millions of investors and potential investors.

COMPANY EARNINGS

Three things happen with the earnings from a company. First, it can be retained by the company in order to help the company grow. The company might build new stores or new factories. It might pay off debt. It might spend it on research and development. It might simply buff up its cash reserves for a rainy day. Each of these adds value to the company, hopefully more than the cost of the investment.

Second, the company can simply distribute cash to its owners. This is known as a dividend. The owners can use the dividend to buy more shares of the company if they wish, but they can also use it to invest in something else (adding diversification), or even just spend the money on their own living expenses.

Third, the company may buy back its own shares. Remember a company "goes public" (or sells shares) to raise cash for the company or its owners. Buying back shares is just the opposite. This can also be a positive for the investors. Yes, the company is worth less (since it has less cash) but there are also fewer shares (and thus a higher price per share), so the value of an individual investor's holdings actually went up. Many investors prefer this approach to receiving dividends. At least in a taxable account, investors are taxed on any distributed dividends, whether they want to take money out of the investment or not. But that is not the case with share buy-backs, since no income was distributed to the investor.

Thus the less of a company's earnings that is paid out to the investors (and thus taxed), the more tax-efficient the investment. If a company does not pay out any dividends, the investor will pay no taxes on its earnings until selling the shares. In fact, if the investor dies before selling them, those earnings will not be subject to income tax at all due to the step-up in basis. That means that when the investor's heirs go to sell their inherited investment, the IRS considers them to have bought it at the price on the day of the investor's death, and they only have to pay capital gains taxes on the difference between the value on the day they sell and the value on the day the investor died. That can be a huge difference from the tax bill due if the investor sold the investment before dying.

While dividends are a nice demonstration that the company is indeed profitable, tax considerations aside, an investor should be agnostic as to whether the earnings are paid out as dividends, used for share buybacks, or reinvested in the company. If the company can use the earnings to grow faster than the overall market, it should retain them. If the shares are trading for less than the company feels they are worth it should use excess cash to buy shares back. If neither of these are true, the company should distribute dividends.

UNDERSTANDING THE STOCK MARKET

I hope walking through this exercise demonstrates to you that when you own shares of stock you own real, live companies. They have real assets, employ real people, and earn real money. So while it is obviously possible to lose money in the stock market, investing in these companies for the long run is hardly the casino its critics claim the stock market to be.

The problem is that if you were to watch the day-to-day movements of the stock market, it would feel like a casino. The value of a company might go up 5 or 10% in a year, but the route to get there will be anything but smooth. In fact, the company might lose or gain 5–10% a day many times during that year. Benjamin Graham famously described the market as a voting machine in the short term, but a weighing machine in the long run.[44] A great deal of the volatility you see in stock prices is due to a speculative component. Investors may be wildly optimistic about the prospects for the overall economy or a single company one day, and then incredibly pessimistic the next. None of that has any effect on the actual earnings of a company though, and over the long run, the optimism and pessimism will cancel each other out. The value of the company will come only from its earnings and how well it can grow those earnings.

It is the same for a rental property. Just like a stock trades with a certain P/E ratio, a given property "trades" (although much more infrequently and with greater expenses) at a capitalization rate. A "cap rate" might be 6. That means that after collecting all revenue (usually all or mostly rent) and paying all non-mortgage expenses (such as management fees, maintenance, property taxes, and insurance), the cash flow left over for the owner is 6% of the value of the property. If the property continues to be valued at a cap rate of 6%, the only way for it to become more valuable is for it to increase its earnings. However, cap rates can change. When a cap rate increases, it is because the owner and potential owners think its prospects of increasing its earnings have gone down and vice versa. Cap rates may also change if alternative investments become more or less attractive in comparison.

If you wish to be a successful investor, do not get caught up in the speculative elements of your productive assets. If P/E ratios go up or cap rates fall, that should just be icing on the cake. Assume the speculative component of your investments will remain stable and focus on the earnings and how likely they are to grow.

It is important to understand the difference between return and yield. The total return is the return on your investment. For a stock, that is the increase (or decrease) in price plus the dividends. If the stock had a dividend of 2% and increased in price 7% over the course of a year, its total return over that year was 9%. Its yield, however, was 2%. Yield is the income paid out by an investment.

A mutual fund or rental property works the same way. A rental property, at least a paid off one, often has a higher yield than a typical stock or mutual fund. Perhaps a paid-off, cap rate 6 property pays a yield of 6%. If it also appreciated 3% in value, then the total return would be 9%. It is critical to understand the difference between yield and return and to focus on the total return. The problem with focusing on just yield is that it can lead you to purchase investments with a poor total return despite an exceptional yield.

Yield vs. Return

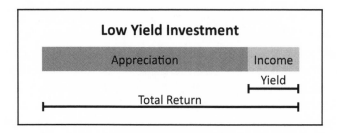

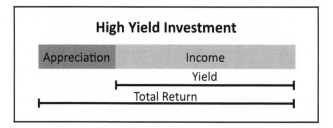

A perfect example of this might be peer to peer loans, which are unsecured loans made to individuals. This loan might carry an interest rate of 20% (the yield) but since 10–30% of borrowers eventually default on the loans, the total return will be much lower than 20%, and perhaps even negative. Likewise, the stocks of many companies that are in dire straits may report very high yields. It is important to understand what they are actually reporting. For example, if they are reporting a "trailing dividend yield," they are dividing the last dividend it paid by the current value of the company. If the company has just had a dramatic decrease in value due to some new development or economic situation, that trailing dividend yield will look very high. A company might also report a "forward dividend yield," the expected dividends in the next year divided by the current value of the company. That might seem more accurate, until you realize that it requires predicting the future. Each type of yield has its pros and cons, but it is important to realize the implications of each. A mutual fund typically reports only its trailing yield over the last 12 months, often calling it a "distribution yield."

Another term you will hear thrown around regarding the stock market is market capitalization. This is a fancy word that simply describes the size of a company. A "mega-cap" or "large-cap" is a big company, with billions of dollars in earnings. There is no set cut-off, but these companies are typically worth $10 billion or more. All of the companies in the Dow Jones index and most of the companies in the S&P 500 index are large-cap companies. These are the companies you have heard of, including Microsoft, Amazon, Facebook, Apple, Alphabet (Google), Exxon, General Electric, etc.

Further divisions include mid-cap stocks ($2–$10 billion), small-cap stocks ($300 million–$2 billion), and micro-cap stocks ($50–$300 million). While it would still be pretty awesome to own a company worth "just $20–$30 million," keep in mind we are discussing publicly traded companies, meaning companies that got so big that they really can only be owned by thousands of people. There just are not that many people in the world who actually have $20 million that are willing to put it into a single company. The smaller the company, the riskier the investment tends to be. This increased risk should lead to higher expected returns. An investor should logically demand to have a higher return in order to invest in a company with only a single product or that is highly dependent on a few key people. Sometimes that additional return "premium" shows up and sometimes it does not, but on average over decades, smaller stocks have had higher returns than larger stocks.

Equity Style Box

STYLE

SIZE	Value	Blend	Growth
Large Cap	Large Value	Large Blend	Large Growth
Mid Cap	Mid Value	Mid Blend	Mid Growth
Small Cap	Small Value	Small Blend	Small Growth

Besides market capitalization, the stock market is also often divided up by valuation metrics or investing style. There are numerous valuation metrics including the aforementioned Price to Earnings Ratio. These include dividend yield, Price to Book (P/B) Ratio, Price to Sales (P/S) Ratio, and Price to Cash Flow (P/CF). The basic theory is the same though. Some companies are expected to grow quickly and thus trade at high P/E, P/B, P/S, P/CF ratios and low dividend yields. These are called "growth" stocks, and it can be exciting to own them. If people are talking about stocks around the water cooler, they are likely naming only growth stocks.

On the other end of the spectrum are companies with low ratios and high dividend yields. These tend to be boring, stodgy companies that have been around a long-time, have stable cash-flow, and have limited growth prospects. These are called "value" stocks. You can buy a dollar of earnings for a much lower price when you buy a value stock than when you buy a growth stock. If people become too pessimistic about the prospects of a value stock or too optimistic about the prospects of a growth stock (as they often do), the value stock can end up with a higher return, even though the company is growing at a slower rate! In fact, over the decades, the data has been pretty clear that value stocks outperform growth stocks over the long run. However, just like with large and small-cap stocks, it might take a very long time for you to receive that "premium."

Since the overall stock market is composed primarily of large growth stocks, any time your own portfolio has more small stocks and value stocks in it than the overall market does, you will have "tracking error" when comparing the returns of your portfolio to those of the overall market. It can be very difficult behaviorally to stay the course with your investing plan when you are trailing the overall market for years or even a decade or more, so if you decide to "tilt" your portfolio toward small and value stocks, be certain you do not tilt it more than you can tolerate even if those premiums do not show up for years and years.

Portfolio analysts love to use a tic-tac-toe style box made famous by a company called Morningstar to demonstrate the tilts of a portfolio. On the X-axis, you see a continuum of Value to Growth (often with "Blend" in the middle) and on the Y-axis you see a continuum of Mega-Cap down to Micro-Cap. This allows you to see where a stock, mutual fund, or even your entire stock portfolio falls in the marketplace and is a handy way to think about the stock market.

In addition to market capitalization and style of investing, the market is also divided into 11 sectors. Each sector describes a certain type of company that makes money in a certain way. The sectors are further divided into 2–11 industries each. Here are the various sectors, their relative size as of January 2020, the number of industries in each sector, and some representative companies.[45]

Stock Market Divided by Sectors			
Sector	Size	Industries	Examples of Companies
Communication Services	$5.5 trillion	5	AT&T. Verizon
Consumer Discretionary	$5.9 trillion	11	Amazon, Home Depot, McDonalds, Nike
Consumer Staples	$4.1 trillion	6	Wal-mart, Proctor & Gamble, Coca-Cola
Energy	$3.3 trillion	2	Exxon, Chevron
Financials	$7.5 trillion	7	Berkshire-Hathaway, Bank of America
Healthcare	$6.3 trillion	6	Johnson & Johnson, Pfizer
Industrials	$4.6 trillion	14	Boeing, Union Pacific
Information Technology	$9.6 trillion	6	Apple, Microsoft
Materials	$2.0 trillion	5	Rio Tinto, International Paper
Real Estate	$1.4 trillion	2	Brookfield, Simon Property, Zillow
Utilities	$1.6 trillion	5	Dominion Energy, Exelon

As you can see, the stocks in the overall stock market can be divided lots of different ways and endlessly studied by those with the interest. Whether the time and effort that goes into that study will pay off with higher returns is an entirely different question. Stock investing can actually be incredibly simple. You can just buy all of the stocks using a "Total Stock Market" index fund. You will own all the growth stocks, all the value stocks, all the large stocks, all the small stocks, and every stock in every sector and industry. So if you are finding that you really do not care about this stuff, good news! You do not have to in order to be a successful investor!

INTEREST-BEARING INVESTMENTS (BONDS)

Let us turn now briefly to the subject of bonds. If stocks and real estate are the sports cars of your portfolio, bonds are the pick-up trucks and minivans: practical, but not very exciting. Stocks, with their higher long-term returns, allow you to eat well in retirement. Bonds, with their lower volatility, allow you to sleep well.

A lot of people find bonds to be very confusing, which is surprising to me as I find them far easier to understand than stocks. Part of the problem seems to be that people simply do not understand the terminology of a bond. Remember a bond is simply a loan to a company or government. The company has to pay the bondholder a certain dividend every so often, typically quarterly, and then after the term of the bond is up (the bond "matures") the company must pay the principal back to the bondholder. When the bond is issued, its yield is often called a "coupon" or "coupon yield." That is because bonds used to have a little coupon physically attached to them that you would break off and turn in to get your dividend. The coupons are long gone in our computer age, but the term has stuck around.

Once a bond is issued, however, its yield is no longer the same as the coupon yield. That is because of the two main risks of bonds—interest rate risk and credit risk. If you can simply understand these two risks, you can understand 99% of what you need to know about bonds and the mutual funds that invest in them.

Interest rate risk is the risk that interest rates go up. The price of a bond is inversely correlated to interest rates. If interest rates go up after a bond is issued, the price falls. If interest rates go down, the price rises. This is completely logical, of course. If you have a bond with a coupon of 5% and interest rates suddenly go up to 6%, why would anyone want your bond when they can just go out and buy a new one that pays 6% instead of 5%? They would not. So in order to entice someone to buy your bond, you have to discount the price. How much do you have to discount it? Just enough so that the yield on your bond is also equal to 6%. The company, of course, is still paying that coupon yield, 5% of the original price of the bond each year. And when the term of the bond is up, it is still obligated to give you back your principal. Thus, the closer you get to the day when the company will pay back your principal, the less changes in interest rates matter. Interest rate risk is often called term risk. The longer the time period (term) until the company pays back the principal, the more sensitive the bond is to changes in interest rates.

A measurement of the sensitivity of a bond (or collection of bonds) to interest rates is called duration. Duration is measured in years. Perhaps the easiest way to think of duration is how many years at the new higher yield it will take for a bond to make up for loss in value caused by a 1% increase in interest rates. Duration is never longer than the maturity of the bond.

Term risk (or interest rate risk) is generally divided into long-term bonds (10–30 years), intermediate-term bonds (2–10 years), and short-term bonds (<2 years). The decision of whether to take on additional term risk basically rests on three factors. The first is whether you think interest rates are going to go down, remain stable, or go up. If rates go down, the value of the bonds will increase—the longer the duration the better. If rates remain stable, the higher interest rates generally paid by longer bonds will provide higher returns. If interest rates rise, however, the longer-term bonds will lose the most value, at least for any period of time shorter than the duration. So if you believe you can predict future interest rates, you should choose your bonds accordingly. This is obviously somewhat speculative and if you peer into your crystal ball and honestly have no idea what interest rates are going to do (which is likely correct), this is a factor that should probably be ignored.

The second factor is your time horizon for this money. One nice thing about high-quality bonds, at least if bought individually, is that at the end of the term you get your principal back. Changes in bond value do not actually matter if you hold the bond until it matures. So one safe option is simply to buy a bond that matures about the time that you need the money. Need money in 5 years? Buy a five-year bond. That may be a bit over-conservative, but as a general rule, you want to keep the average duration of your bond portfolio shorter than your need for the money. If you do that, when interest rates rise you will have sufficient time for the additional yield to make up for the loss of principal caused by rising rates.

The third factor is how much you are compensated for taking on additional term risk. A long-term bond should offer a much higher yield than a short-term bond in order to entice you to take on that risk. Only you can decide how much compensation is enough. There are some rules of thumb out there, perhaps the most common being to make sure you get 0.20% in extra yield for every year of extra duration, but those rules can break down at very high or very low interest rates. Since current yield is generally the best predictor of future returns with bonds, you want to make sure you are being paid to take on additional risk. Yield curves can flatten (meaning a long-term bond does not have a higher yield than a short-term bond) or even invert (meaning a short-term bond has a higher yield than a long-term bond). These events have some correlation with economic and stock downturns, but from a bond only perspective, the only reason an investor would "go long" in those situations is if the investor is convinced interest rates will soon fall.

Now we will turn to credit risk. Up until this point, we have assumed that if you buy a bond, essentially loaning your money to a company or government, that the borrower is actually good for it. That is not necessarily the case. Sometimes a borrower only pays back part of a loan or defaults on it completely. This is known as credit risk. The more credit risk you take on, the higher a yield you should demand. There are rating agencies that rate bond issuers. While each agency has its own scale, it is generally the same as buying eggs or earning grades in high school. As are better than Bs, and Bs are better than Cs. These agencies rate national governments, state and municipal governments, corporations, and even asset-based bonds such as mortgage-backed bonds.

Debt Style Box

DURATION

	Short	Medium	Long
High	High Short	High Medium	High Long
Medium	Medium Short	Medium Medium	Medium Long
Low	Low Short	Low Medium	Low Long

CREDIT QUALITY

As a general rule, US treasuries are considered the safest bonds—the least likely to default. Only slightly behind are municipal bonds, issued by states and municipalities. Each of these entities has the ability to tax millions of taxpayers to pay its obligations, a substantial advantage over a corporation. Thus, corporate bonds are considered more likely to default. As the bond rating for a corporation falls, eventually it falls into "junk bond territory," typically ratings with Bs and Cs in them. Just like you generally get a higher yield for taking on more term risk (longer bonds), you also generally get a higher yield for taking on additional credit risk. Thus, junk bonds yield more than corporate bonds yield more than treasury bonds. Theoretically, your total return on the bond should also be higher, but that depends on the default rate. In good times when there are few defaults, the higher yield of a junk bond is likely to result in a higher return than the lower yield of a treasury bond. When defaults rise in bad economic times, the higher yield may not be able to make up for all of those defaults.

This is often seen as a "flight to quality" in an economic downturn, when the highest quality bonds, generally treasury bonds, rise the most in value while lower quality bonds rise less or even fall in value. Due to this effect, it is critical to not "chase yield," meaning invest in an investment just because the yield is high without considering the total return or how the investment might interact with the rest of your portfolio. Once more, there is a spread between corporate bonds and treasury bonds, and you want to make sure you are being adequately compensated with a higher yield in order to take on that credit risk. How much is enough extra yield? It is hard to say, but keep in mind that the spread between corporate bond yields and treasury yields of bonds of the same maturity has varied between 1.6% and 6% over the last 20 years, generally hanging out in the 2–3% range.

Municipal bonds are a bit of a special case. Federal income taxes do not apply to the interest from these bonds, and you generally do not pay state income taxes on bonds issued in your state. Thus, investors in a high tax bracket who buy their bonds outside of a tax-protected retirement account may discover that a municipal bond actually offers a higher after-tax yield for them. Due to this effect, municipal bonds generally offer a lower interest rate than fully taxable bonds, saving states and cities money while still offering an attractive investment for well-heeled investors.

Another unique type of bond is an inflation-indexed bond, such as Treasury Inflation Protected Security or TIPS. One of the biggest risks to your bond portfolio is rapidly rising inflation, especially since it is often accompanied by a rapid rise in interest rates. Even moderate inflation can be devastating to a bond portfolio. Inflation-indexed bonds help protect you from unexpected inflation. With a normal or "nominal" bond, your return comes from two places—the yield and the change in value of the bond as interest rates or credit quality changes. With an inflation-indexed bond, there is a third source of return, an inflation adjustment that is periodically applied. That means these bonds have a lower return if inflation is lower than expected, but will have a higher return if inflation rises. This protection is attractive to many investors who include both nominal and inflation-indexed bonds in their portfolio. Similar protection is available with I bonds, a type of US Savings Bond.

Wow! Did that section about bonds put you to sleep or what? Boring! The good news is that you now know more about bonds than most who call themselves financial advisors. The even better news? You do not have to remember any of that stuff. Just remember that when you want some bonds in your portfolio all you have to remember is to buy a low-cost, broadly diversified bond mutual fund such as the Total Bond Market Index Fund from a company like Vanguard or Fidelity.

MUTUAL FUNDS

In fact, mutual funds are the investing vehicle preferred by most informed investors and nearly all retirement funds. Remember a mutual fund offers several advantages over purchasing individual securities like stocks and bonds:

- Professional Management
- Daily Liquidity
- Economies of Scale
- Diversification

While there are thousands of mutual funds out there, selecting appropriate funds for your portfolio is actually relatively easy. As discussed earlier, over the long run low-cost index funds are highly likely to outperform most actively managed funds, especially if you are investing outside of a tax-protected retirement account. Thus, right off the bat you can essentially cross all of the actively managed mutual funds off your list. If you will also avoid the high-cost index funds that exist and the niche, gimmicky funds, you will find that you are really only choosing between a few dozen index funds from a handful of fund companies who all offer a collection of almost identical funds. This phenomenon makes selecting investments incredibly easy.

For example, perhaps you have decided that you want to invest a portion of your portfolio into US Stocks. Since you know index funds are a smart way to invest, you look for a broadly diversified index fund that invests in US stocks. These are usually called Total Stock Market Index Funds or something similar. If you look at all of these and then sort for price (called the expense ratio of the mutual fund), you will discover that the lowest cost funds are offered by companies like Vanguard, Fidelity, Charles Schwab, and iShares. Each has a fund that costs almost nothing that simply buys all of the stocks in the US in proportion to the overall market. The differences between these funds are trivial and you can safely invest in any of them.

Before purchasing a mutual fund, it is important to know what you are investing in. Each mutual fund is required to provide a standardized prospectus which will tell you what it invests in. Vanguard does a particularly nice job of putting together a straightforward prospectus. The investment strategy and investment policy of the Vanguard Total Stock Market Funds reads as follows:

> "The Fund employs an indexing investment approach designed to track the performance of the CRSP US Total Market Index, which represents approximately 100% of the investable U.S. stock market and includes large-, mid-, small-, and micro-cap stocks regularly traded on the New York Stock Exchange and Nasdaq. The fund invests by sampling the Index, meaning that it holds a broadly diversified collection of securities that, in the aggregate, approximates the full Index in terms of key characteristics. These key characteristics include industry weightings and market capitalization, as well as certain financial measures, such as price/earnings ratio and dividend yield."[46]

As you can see, the fund simply tries to obtain the return of the index, or the overall market and will invest almost entirely in US stocks. Now, you can turn to the track record of the fund to make sure that it actually does this. You will find that later in the prospectus. For this particular fund, you can see that from the end of 2009 to the end of 2019, the fund had an annualized return of 13.42% and the index it was tracking had a return of 13.44%. So yes, you can see that the fund managers are doing a fine job of tracking the index. You can also lookup the expenses of the fund. Some mutual funds have all kinds of expenses such as loads (commissions) and 12b-1 (marketing) fees. You will want to avoid any fund with either of those fees.

However, every fund has expenses that are passed on to the investors. These are reported in a standard way called an expense ratio—the percentage of the fund assets that go toward the expenses of the fund each year. The average for all mutual funds is about 1% per year, but that would be ridiculously high for a large, broadly diversified index mutual fund. If you are paying more than 0.2% for one of those funds, you are paying too much. Typical expense ratios for the index funds from the best companies range from 0.00 to 0.10% these days. That means for every $10,000 you have invested, you will be paying $0–$10 in fees. Essentially free. Since you can obtain this professional management, diversification, and liquidity for almost nothing, it makes little sense for you to try to do this on your own by picking your own stocks and bonds.

A portfolio is simply a collection of investments. "My portfolio" is simply a fancy term that means "all of my investments." Speaking the language of finance not only keeps you from looking like an uneducated sucker, but allows you to have precise discussions just like you are used to in medicine. Stocks, bonds, and mutual funds are the basic investments that make up the majority of the portfolios of most investors. These are generally considered "traditional" investments. Anything else is considered to be a non-traditional or "alternative" investment. Traditional investments are the best studied, best understood, and most widely available. That does not necessarily mean there is no role for alternative investments in your portfolio, but it does behoove you to at least understand how traditional investments work as you become financially literate.

There! You made it to the end of this chapter. Was that so bad? You might not yet realize it, but you now know more than 90% of your peers about this subject and more than quite a few people who call themselves "financial advisors." As the years go by and compound interest starts to work on your savings, the value of the knowledge you just acquired in this chapter will grow to far more than anything else you have read this year. Sorry it was so boring.

MAIN IDEAS

- Financial literacy is extremely valuable information, particularly to a high-earning doctor or dentist.

- Finance has a language all its own, just like medicine, where the terms have precise meanings.

- Stocks represent real ownership in a publicly traded company. When the company makes money, you make money.

- The value of a stock is dependent on the estimated future earnings of the company.

- Bonds are a loan to a government or company. While they have lower expected long-term returns than stocks, they are also much less volatile and less subject to loss.

- Bond prices and interest rates are inversely correlated.

- Mutual funds are composed of the pooled investments of many investors. They provide diversification, liquidity, pooled costs, and professional management.

- Low-cost, broadly diversified index funds are an ideal component of a retirement portfolio.

ADDITIONAL RESOURCES

- **Online Course:** Fire Your Financial Advisor
whitecoatinvestor.teachable.com/p/fire-your-financial-advisor

- **Blog Post:** Investing 101
www.whitecoatinvestor.com/investing-101/

- **Blog Post:** You Need an Investing Plan
  www.whitecoatinvestor.com/investing/you-need-an-investing-plan/

- **Blog Post:** Why Talking About Individual Stocks (and Sectors) Makes You Look Dumb
  www.whitecoatinvestor.com/individual-stocks-dumb/

- **Blog Post:** 7 Basic Principles of Bond Investing
  www.whitecoatinvestor.com/bonds-back-to-basics/

- **Blog Post:** 7 Reasons Not to Use a 100% Stock Portfolio
  www.whitecoatinvestor.com/100-stock-portfolio/

- **Blog Post:** 150 Portfolios Better than Yours
  www.whitecoatinvestor.com/150-portfolios-better-than-yours/

- **Blog Post:** 10 Reasons I Invest in Index Funds
  www.whitecoatinvestor.com/10-reasons-invest-index-funds/

- **Blog Post:** Why Does the Stock Market Go Up?
  www.whitecoatinvestor.com/why-does-the-stock-market-go-up/

CHAPTER TWENTY

TAXES AND RETIREMENT ACCOUNTS

(FINANCIAL LITERACY 102)

Another important aspect of becoming financially literate is understanding the tax code and its interactions with your financial life. While nobody has ever actually read the entire tax code (the Internal Revenue Code is over 6,500 pages and there are over 60,000 pages of associated case law), a basic understanding of how taxes on income work is critical to becoming financially literate. Perhaps the most important aspect of the tax code for high-income professionals is the variety of tax-protected accounts designed to pay for retirement, health care, and education.

In this chapter, we will go over the basics of the tax code with a special focus on tax-protected accounts. Unfortunately, the tax code is constantly changing, which will make this chapter out of date in some way before you even read it. Because of this, I will endeavor to paint mostly in broad strokes so that your knowledge of taxes will be a bit more evergreen. Recognize that there will be subtle and not so subtle changes every year, particularly to contribution amounts for each type of account. Of course, if you are not located in the United States, only a minimal amount of this chapter will be useful to you. I would encourage you to spend some time studying the tax laws of your own country.

Income taxes in the United States are levied by the federal government, most state governments, and even some local governments. In this chapter, I will primarily focus on the federal income tax. Not only would a chapter discussing laws from over 40 states be painfully long, but federal taxes are generally the lion's share of your tax burden even if you live in a state with relatively high tax rates. The US Income Tax is far younger than the Republic and actually has a pretty interesting history. For the first 100 years of the Republic, the federal government was primarily funded by tariffs. There was an income tax from 1862 to 1871 and then growing political pressure from populists increased as the century went on. It was felt that tariffs, like a sales tax, unfairly placed the burden of funding the government on the poor. In 1894, an income tax provision was passed by Congress. However, in a famous court case (Pollock v. Farmer's Loan & Trust Co.) it was struck down as unconstitutional in 1895. Our system of checks and balances allows for the constitution to change, and so it was with the sixteenth amendment ratified in 1913. Since that time we have had a progressive income tax.

Compared to today's tax burden, the 1913 income tax seems downright trivial. The first tax bracket, including the first $20,000 of taxable income ($523,000 in 2020 dollars) was just 1%. One did not enter the top tax bracket of 7% until an income of $500,000 ($13,081,000 in 2020 dollars). Since that time, the tax rates have gone up and down and become more and less progressive depending on which political party was in power. At one point, the highest marginal tax bracket was over 90%, although that only applied to a very small number of people, which brings us to our first critical tax concept for you to understand.

INCOME TAX BRACKETS

A marginal tax rate is that rate at which the last dollar you earn is taxed. This number is also often referred to as your tax bracket. However, it does not mean that all of your income is taxed at that rate. Only the amount of money in your top bracket is taxed at your marginal tax rate. Thus, when the tax brackets are applied to your income, your income fills each bracket as it goes along. In 2021, the tax brackets are as follows:[47] *(found in the table at the tops of the next page)*.

Since a good chunk of your income will be taxed at 10, 12, 22, or 24%, someone with a marginal tax rate of 32% will have an effective tax rate of much less than 32%. This becomes especially true once you consider the effect of deductions such as the standard deduction and contributions to tax-deferred retirement accounts. In fact, our tax code is so progressive, that over 40% of taxpayers pay no federal income taxes at all (once all deductions and credits are considered), 39% of federal income taxes are paid by the top 1% (hopefully soon to be you), and 70% of taxes are paid by the top 10%.

2021 Federal Income Tax Brackets		
Tax Rate	Taxable Income Single	Taxable Income Married Filing Jointly
10%	$0–$9,950	$0–$19,900
12%	$9,951–$40,525	$19,901–$81,050
22%	$40,526–$86,375	$81,051–$172,750
24%	$86,376–$164,925	$172,751–$329,850
32%	$164,926–$209,425	$329,851–$418,850
35%	$209,426–$523,600	$418,851–$623,300
37%	>$523,600	>$623,300

Politics aside, the critical concept for you to understand is that your marginal tax rate is not your effective tax rate. Both numbers are important and are worth calculating each year, however. So while the top tax bracket has been over 90% back in the 1940s, 1950s, and 1960s,[48] the effective tax rate on the top 1% of earners in the US has been pretty consistently between 32% and 46% since World War II.[49]

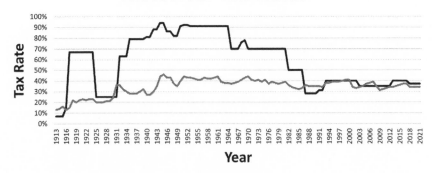

Historical Tax Rates

——Top Federal Marginal Income Tax Rate

——Effective Tax Rate on Top 1% (Includes Federal, State, and Local Taxes)

CRITICAL CONCEPTS

The US Tax Code is primarily run on the honor system. While the Internal Revenue Service (IRS) does perform audits on a small percentage of returns each year, most of those audits are automated and are simply comparing the numbers you put on your return with the numbers reported on the returns of others, such as your employer.

The federal tax system is a pay as you go system, so you are expected to pay as you earn the money. Employers are required to withhold taxes from your paychecks and submit that money to the government on your behalf. The self-employed are required to make quarterly estimated tax payments.

The second critical tax concept for you to understand is that the amount of money withheld (or paid in estimated payments) is only somewhat related to how much money you actually owe. It is possible that the amount of money your employer is required to withhold from your paycheck is an amount that is either significantly larger or significantly smaller than your actual tax bill. Each April 15th you are required to file a tax return and at that point, you and the IRS settle up. If you paid too much, the IRS sends you a refund. If you paid too little, you send the IRS a check.

Many naive taxpayers actually get excited to receive a tax refund check. They oddly use it as a sort of Christmas Club savings account, and then use the lump sum they receive after filing their tax return to pay bills, buy a car, or go on a vacation. In reality, all they did was provide an interest-free loan to the government. If you find that you are getting large tax refunds, you may be able to adjust your withholdings with your employer (using Form W-4) to have less tax withheld from each paycheck.

Ideally, you get an interest-free loan from the government. The truly savvy attempt to pay as little as possible before their tax due date. Of course, you do not want to pay too little, or you will owe a penalty, and naturally, you want to make sure you still have the money to pay the taxes when they become due.

The process of matching estimated tax payments to actual taxes due is even trickier for the self-employed such as an independent contractor or practice owner. At a minimum, they want to make sure they pay enough in advance to be in the "safe harbor," where no penalty will be assessed. For a high earner, that safe harbor is either paying 100% of taxes due (within

$1,000) or at least 110% of what was due on last year's tax return. Thus an easy way for a self-employed doctor to calculate their quarterly estimated tax payments is to multiply their tax bill from the year before by 110% and then divide by four. Note that that figure has absolutely nothing to do with your income from this year or your tax bill for this year. It is possible to pay way too much or way too little using this method and you will need to settle up when you file your tax return.

THE INCOME TAX RETURN

The tax return assists you in calculating your tax bill. The basic process is to first add up all your sources of income. These include salaries, profits from businesses you own, rents from rental properties, dividends, interest, and royalties. This gives you your total income. Next you subtract "above the line" deductions from this income. This includes contributions to retirement accounts, health insurance premiums for the self-employed, HSA contributions, alimony paid, student loan interest for low earners, and tuition paid. This leaves you with your "adjusted gross income" (AGI). The AGI line on your tax form is "the line" they are talking about when they talk about "above the line" and "below the line" deductions. The AGI is a figure that is used throughout the tax code and with numerous government benefits.

Next you apply either the standard deduction ($12,550 single, $25,100 married filing jointly for 2021) or, for a small percentage of taxpayers who are usually high earners, you itemize your below the line deductions. These include up to $10,000 in state/local income taxes or property taxes, charitable contributions, and home mortgage interest. Rarely, people can also deduct some medical expenses and losses due to disasters and theft here.

Once you apply either the standard deduction or your itemized deductions (whichever is larger), you are left with your taxable income. Your total tax bill for the year is then calculated from this number using the tax brackets.

Following this calculation, any tax credits you qualify for are applied. A tax credit is even better than a tax deduction. A deduction is simply a portion of your income on which taxes are not calculated. A credit is actually a dollar for dollar reduction in your tax bill. If your marginal tax rate is 25%, a $1,000 tax credit is worth four times as much as a $1,000 tax deduction, which is only worth $250. Some tax credits are even refundable, meaning you can have a negative tax bill, but most are non-refundable and thus will not reduce your tax bill below $0. The most common refundable tax credits, the earned income tax credit and the child tax credit, are available to many medical and dental students. Once tax credits are subtracted from your tax, you can then apply any money withheld by employers or paid as a quarterly estimated payment. If you still owe money, you write a check. If you have overpaid, you will receive a refund.

Once you understand this framework, everything else about the tax code can be hung in the proper place on the framework.

Total Income -

Above the line deductions =

Adjusted Gross Income (AGI)

Adjusted Gross Income (AGI) -

Below the line deductions =

Taxable income

Taxable income x

Tax rate(s) =

Tax

Tax -

Tax Credits -

Taxes already paid =

Tax due with the return

Let us do a quick example to demonstrate. Let us say a single independent contractor physician earns $200,000 after paying all business expenses. So total income is $200,000. The doc contributed $40,000 to a retirement account and $5,000 to a health savings account, both above the line deductions. That left the doctor with an adjusted gross income of $155,000. The doctor gave $8,000 to charity, paid over $10,000 in state and property taxes, and paid $18,000 in mortgage interest. Since the total of $8,000 + $10,000 + $18,000 = $36,000 and $36,000 is more than the standard deduction, this physician chooses to itemize deductions instead of taking the standard deduction. That leaves the doctor with $155,000 - $36,000 = $119,000 in taxable income.

In 2021, this doctor will pay the following amounts in tax on a taxable income of $119,000.

> First $9,950 x 10% = $995
>
> Next $30,575 x 12% = $3,669
>
> Next $45,850 x 22% = $10,087
>
> Next $32,625 x 24% = $7,830
>
> Total = $22,581

That is an effective tax rate of 19% of $119,000 and 11% of $200,000.

PAYROLL TAXES

In addition to income taxes, your employer will also deduct payroll (or FICA) taxes from your paychecks. The two main payroll taxes are Social Security and Medicare tax. For 2020, Social Security tax is 12.4% of your first $142,800 of salary income, or a total of $17,707. If you are an employee, your employer will pay half of that amount. If you are self-employed, you will be responsible for both halves, but will be able to deduct the employer half. This is often called "Self-Employment Tax" but is just another name for payroll taxes. Medicare tax is 2.9% of all salary income. Unlike Social Security tax, there is no wage limit above which you do not owe Medicare taxes. Again, half of this tax is paid by the employer if you are an employee, but you pay both halves of it if you are self-employed (but can deduct the employer half as an above the line deduction).

Many high earners also pay "Additional Medicare Tax." This is an additional 0.9% tax paid by the employee on any earned income (salary or self-employment income) above a modified adjusted gross income of $200,000 ($250,000 Married Filing Jointly). This tax was added in 2014 as part of the Patient Protection and Affordable Care Act. If employed, your employer will withhold this on your behalf. The self-employed will pay it as part of their self-employment tax. Additional Medicare Tax, like the federal income tax, is a progressive tax, since only high earners pay it. Medicare tax is a flat tax, since everybody pays the same percentage of their income no matter how much they make. Social Security tax is actually a regressive tax, since it is not applied above the Social Security wage limit ($142,800 in 2021). Social Security benefits are still quite progressive however since the "return" on your "investment" becomes lower as you pay more in Social Security tax.

There is a quirk regarding Social Security tax when you have multiple employers. Each employer must withhold it on the first $142,800 (2021) in wages, even if you have two or three employers. You can apply to have the employee half refunded to you with your tax return, but the employer cannot. This is true even if one of your employers is a corporation entirely owned by you. Thus many high earners with multiple jobs find it beneficial to make sure only one of them is an employee job.

Income is divided between earned income and unearned income. The difference is that payroll taxes are only calculated on earned income, like salary income and most types of self-employment income. However, you do not have to pay payroll taxes on unearned income such as interest, dividends, some royalties, rents, capital gains, or S Corporation distributions. For this reason, some doctors form an S Corp and split their income between salary and distributions, saving themselves a few thousand dollars a year in Medicare taxes. The IRS requires them to pay a reasonable salary for the work done, of course. A salary of $30,000 and a distribution of $300,000 is not going to be viewed as reasonable for a doctor.

QUALIFIED DIVIDEND AND LONG-TERM CAPITAL GAINS TAX RATES

Investment income can also be taxed at a lower rate. If you have held an investment for at least a year before selling it for a gain, it qualifies for the lower long-term capital gains tax rates, which range from 0–20%, much lower than the 10–37% brackets used for ordinary income. This is one reason why day traders generally underperform long-term, buy-and-hold investors—their tax costs are much higher. Qualified dividends also qualify for these same lower tax rates. Qualified dividends generally must be paid by a corporation in the US or a country with whom the US has a tax treaty and you must have held the stock for at least 60 days. Note that bond dividends generally are not qualified. Like other investment income, long-term capital gains and qualified dividends are susceptible to a 3.8% "Net Investment Income Tax" for those with a modified adjusted gross income over $200,000 ($250,000 Married Filing Jointly). This tax was also part of the Patient Protection and Affordable Care Act put into place in 2014.

199A DEDUCTION

One of the most significant deductions for high earners is the pass-thru income deduction, or 199A deduction, first available in 2018 as part of the Tax Cuts and Jobs Act (TCJA), and scheduled to expire in 2025. The purpose of this deduction was to put pass-thru entities like sole proprietorships, partnerships, S Corporations and Limited Liability Companies taxed as one of the above on a more equal footing with C Corporations, which had their tax rates significantly cut by the TCJA. The deduction can be as large as 20% of your ordinary business income, but can be complicated to actually receive. The biggest issue with this tax deduction as it relates to doctors is that certain businesses, including nearly all high-income professionals like physicians, dentists, attorneys, and accountants, are specifically excluded from this deduction. It disappears over a phaseout range between a taxable income of $164,900 and $214,900 ($329,850 and $429,850 married filing jointly) for 2021. Obviously many specialists and those married to other high earners are not going to be able to get their incomes low enough to qualify for this substantial deduction.

RETIREMENT ACCOUNTS

The other large deduction that is available to most doctors is some form of a tax-deferred retirement account. Part of being financially literate is understanding the ins and outs of all of the various types of tax-protected accounts you are eligible for. The remainder of this chapter will be dedicated to this topic since it is so important for doctors.

There are two main types of retirement accounts, tax-free and tax-deferred which are collectively called "tax-protected." You can usually easily distinguish between the two because tax-free accounts are also called "Roth" accounts (Roth IRA, Roth 401(k), Roth 403(b), Roth 457(b)) after Senator Roth who implemented Roth IRAs back in the 1990s. A tax-free account is the easier type to understand. Once you contribute money to a tax-free account, it is never taxed again. Most investments produce some type of income such as interest, dividends, or capital gains distributions. Inside a tax-protected account of any type, these income distributions are not taxed. This allows the money to grow faster because it is not suffering from a tax drag. Essentially, it has higher returns. A tax-free account enjoys this benefit, but it also benefits from completely tax-free withdrawals. So once you earn money at your job and pay taxes on it, you can then contribute it to a tax-free account where it may grow for many decades tax-free. You will never have to pay taxes on the earnings.

A tax-deferred account, sometimes called a "traditional" retirement account, is slightly more complicated. When you contribute to these accounts, you usually get a deduction equal to the contribution for that tax year. Essentially, you can contribute money to these accounts before it is taxed. This pre-tax money then grows in a tax-protected way, just like in a tax-free account. No tax is due on distributions from your investments inside the account as the money grows over the years. However, when you take the money out of the account, you then must pay taxes on withdrawals at your ordinary income tax rates.

The upfront tax deduction inherent in a tax-deferred account is very useful for doctors, who are usually in one of the highest tax brackets during their peak earnings years. Typically, they are allowed to save tax on the contributed amount entirely at their marginal tax rate. In retirement, they can use the withdrawals to fill the brackets. This usually results in substantial tax rate savings. It would not be unusual for a doctor to save money at 35% and then pay taxes on that money decades later at a rate of 15%. Thus, as a rule of thumb with a few exceptions, high earners should use tax-deferred accounts whenever possible during their peak earnings years. Tax-free accounts should be used in other years (residency, fellowship, sabbaticals, partial retirement) or when tax-deferred accounts are not available. There are exceptions to these rules. For example, the very wealthy should lean toward tax-free accounts and residents going for PSLF should use tax-deferred accounts.

The most well-known retirement account is the 401(k), named after the provision in the tax code that allows for the plan. These plans can be surprisingly complicated. As an employee, you are entitled to be given the 401(k) plan document by your human resources personnel if you ask for it. I suggest you do and then read it. Every plan is a little bit different. The laws allow employees to make either a tax-deferred or tax-free contribution up to $19,500 (2021) per year. If you are 50 or older, you can make an additional $6,500 catch-up contribution, for a total of $26,000. Then the employer may make an additional contribution. The total contribution per 401(k) of employee and employer contributions is $58,000 ($64,500 if 50+) in 2021. If an employee has multiple jobs offering 401(k)s, they are limited to $19,500 ($26,000 if 50+) total into all 401(k)s as an employee contribution. However, the $58,000 ($64,500) limit is per unrelated employer. So with a particularly generous employer, one might be able to get $58,000 into two or even three 401(k)s per year.

The employer contribution typically takes one of three forms. Most common is an employer match. The structure varies, but a common one involves matching 50% of the first 6% of your salary that you put into the 401(k). So if you made $100,000 and you put $6,000 (6%) into the 401(k), your employer would put in $3,000. The second type of employer contribution is a profit-sharing contribution, which is much more common for a high-earner. This is determined by the employer each year and can range from a few thousand dollars to $20,000 or more. Sometimes matches and profit-sharing contributions take several years to "vest," i.e. if you leave the company before they vest, the company keeps their contributions. The third type of contribution is a Qualified Non-Elective Contribution (QNEC), which is always 100% vested. This is a contribution an employer may make in order to remain in compliance with 401(k) laws that prevent the 401(k) from existing solely for the benefit of the owners and/or the most highly paid employees.

When you are a partner in a partnership, you are often allowed to make your own profit-sharing contributions to your 401(k), making it a lot easier to contribute all the way up to the $58,000 (2021) limit each year. The profit-sharing contribution is generally limited to 20% of your net earnings from the partnership. Note that if your business has non-highly compensated employees, they cannot be discriminated against when it comes to the 401(k). There are specific tests that ensure the company owners do not get all of the benefits of the 401(k). Practically speaking, many practice owners find they cannot maximize their 401(k) profit-sharing contribution without making large employer contributions for their employees.

Once the 401(k) contributions are made, the money in the account is invested at your discretion. The usual investment options are mutual funds selected by the employer or their advisor. However, some 401(k)s have a "brokerage window" which allows you to buy any mutual fund you like as well as other investments such as individual stocks and bonds. You can log on to your account and trade these investments every day if you like (although you probably should not do so).

A 403(b) is an account very similar to a 401(k) that is typically available to employees of non-profit institutions such as university physicians. There are a few minor differences, but for nearly all intents and purposes, it functions just like the 401(k) described above.

Both a 401(k) and a 403(b) allow you to withdraw money from them at age 55 without penalty, so long as you are separated from the employer.

A 457(b) is another account frequently available to university physicians. This account differs from a 401(k) or 403(b) in several important ways. First, the money is not technically your money. It is deferred compensation, so it really still belongs to the employer. While this is a good thing in the event that your creditors want access to it, it is a bad thing if your employer's creditors want access to it. So consider carefully the economic stability of your employer before contributing! The second difference is that the withdrawal rules are often unique and certainly different from a typical 401(k) or 403(b). This can be a good thing, in that you can get to your money before age 55 without penalty, but sometimes the withdrawal options are quite limited. Some even make you withdraw the entire account (and pay taxes on it) the year you leave the employer! Be sure the withdrawal options are acceptable to you before contributing. As a general rule, governmental 457(b) plans are better than non-governmental 457(b) plans, because they allow you to roll the money into an IRA when you leave the employer, just like a 401(k) or 403(b). A non-governmental 457(b) does not allow that. The contribution limit to a 457(b) is the same as the employee contribution to a 401(k) or 403(b) ($19,500 in 2021) but the catch-up contributions for those over 50 work slightly differently.

401(k)s, 403(b)s, and 457(b)s are all available with both tax-deferred (traditional) and tax-free (Roth) contributions for the employee contribution. The employer contributions, if any, are always tax-deferred.

Some university employees are also offered a 401(a) plan. 401(a) plans are entirely composed of tax-deferred employer contributions, but you can still control the investments inside.

In addition to these plans offered by employers, every earner (and their spouse) has access to Individual Retirement Arrangements (IRAs) they can purchase on their own, available in both tax-deferred and tax-free flavors, typically from good mutual fund companies or brokerages like Vanguard, Fidelity, Charles Schwab, or eTrade. In 2021, you can contribute $6,000 ($7,000 if 50+) to each spouse's account, even if one spouse is not working. Although IRA fees are usually lower than 401(k) fees and there are more investing options available, IRAs are inferior to 401(k)s in several ways. Contribution limits are obviously lower. In many states, they receive less asset protection from creditors. You also cannot access the funds before age 59 ½ without penalty, although there are exceptions to this rule large enough that you can drive a truck through them. Exceptions include a first home, educational costs (sorry, not student loan payments), and even early retirement so long as you follow a special rule called the Substantially Equal Periodic Payments (SEPP) rule.

Perhaps most importantly, if you are a high earner (phases out at an AGI between $66,000 and $76,000 [$104,000–$124,000 Married Filing Jointly] in 2021) and have a retirement plan available from your employer, you cannot deduct your traditional IRA contributions. You can still make the contributions, you just cannot deduct them. Also, if you have a modified AGI over $125,000–$140,000 ($198,000–$208,000 Married Filing Jointly) in 2021, you cannot make a Roth IRA contribution. There is a workaround to these two rules, however, legal since 2010, called a Backdoor Roth IRA. Since there is no longer an income limit on a Roth conversion (moving money from a traditional IRA to a Roth IRA, paying taxes due if any), many doctors make a non-deductible traditional IRA contribution each year and then subsequently convert it to a Roth IRA. The net effect is the same as contributing directly to a Roth IRA, but it gets you around those pesky income limits.

Self-employed doctors have some other retirement plans available to them. These include a SIMPLE IRA (not the same as a traditional IRA), a SEP-IRA, and a 401(k), often called a solo or individual 401(k) if you have no employees. If you do have employees, choosing between these plans is not a do-it-yourself project, seek reputable assistance. If you do not have employees, the best of these plans to use is almost always an individual 401(k). Many doctors who have an independent contractor (1099) side gig or moonlighting gig will use an individual 401(k) in addition to their regular employee (W-2) job. Contribution limits are the same as for any 401(k). SEP-IRAs are often used by independent contractors, but it is usually a mistake for a doctor to do so. Not only can it require more income to max the account out, but the SEP-IRA, like a traditional IRA, prevents them from doing Backdoor Roth IRAs due to a "pro-rata rule" you need to know about before doing your first Backdoor Roth IRA contribution. There is a tutorial available at *www.whitecoatinvestor.com/backdoor-roth-ira-tutorial/* that explains everything you could ever want to know about the Backdoor

Roth IRA process. If you have two unrelated employers (such as a job as an employee and a moonlighting gig), you can actually use a 401(k) or 403(b) at each of them, although there are a few complicated rules you must follow. You can learn more at *www.whitecoatinvestor.com/multiple-401k-rules/*.

There are two broad categories of retirement plans, defined contribution plans and defined benefit plans. All of the accounts we have discussed above are defined contribution plans. Defined benefits plans are best thought of as pensions, where the employer promises a specific benefit to the employee and all the investment risk in the plan is taken on by the employer instead of the employee (as happens in a 401(k) or an IRA). These traditional pensions are becoming less and less common each year and were never particularly common for doctors. Outside of the military and similar government employers, they are very uncommon these days. However, there is a type of defined benefit plan called a cash balance plan that is much more common among doctors.

The best way to think of a cash balance plan is as an additional 401(k) masquerading as a pension. These are typically put in place by specialist physician partnerships or mid to late-career dentists, but one can even open a personal defined benefit/cash balance plan as an independent contractor. The contribution amounts are actuarially determined and can vary dramatically but often, particularly for older doctors, can be much higher than the 401(k) limits. It is possible to defer as much as $100,000–$200,000 per year into a cash balance plan. If you would like to save more money each year inside tax-deferred retirement accounts than you can fit into your 401(k), look into these plans.

HEALTH SAVINGS ACCOUNTS

Most people do not think of a Health Savings Account (HSA) as a retirement plan, but they should. In 2021, you are eligible to make a $3,600 ($7,200 family) contribution plus a $1,000 catch-up contribution starting at age 55 each year that your only health insurance plan is a High Deductible Health Plan (HDHP). You receive an upfront tax deduction for that contribution, just like a tax-deferred retirement plan. The money grows in a tax-protected way, just like in your retirement accounts. Upon withdrawal, so long as you use it for health care expenses, the money comes out of the account tax-free, just like a Roth IRA or other tax-free account. This triple-tax-free aspect of an HSA makes it the most tax-advantaged investing account out there.

While a health savings account is designed to be used ideally to pay for health care, it can be used for any purpose you like. However, if you use it for something other than health care before age 65, you will have to pay a 20% penalty (and taxes) on the withdrawal. That is a bad idea. However, after age 65, it functions very similarly to any other tax-deferred account in that you only have to pay taxes on the withdrawal. In this way, it functions as a "stealth IRA." Another unique aspect of HSAs is that under current law you do not have to withdraw money from the account in the same year you spend it on health care. You can actually save your receipts for years, allowing the investments in the account to continue to grow before withdrawing money in an amount equal to the receipts tax and penalty-free.

OTHER TAX-PROTECTED ACCOUNTS

Tax-protected accounts are also available for other purposes, including education. The first education accounts were called Coverdell Education Savings Accounts (ESAs). Under current law, you can contribute $2,000 per year per child to these. There is no up-front tax deduction, but they do grow tax-free and so long as the money is used on education, there is no tax bill when the money is withdrawn. Every state also offers a 529 account, with a $15,000 (2021) contribution limit per child. However, the other parent can also open a 529 account for each child if they like. You are also allowed to front-load these accounts for up to five years, so theoretically a couple could put $150,000 into a 529 account for each child in a single year! There is no federal tax deduction for this contribution, but many states allow a deduction or credit for at least part of your contribution. Like an ESA, if the money is used for education it can be withdrawn tax-free. If your state does not offer a special tax break for using their plan, you can use the plan of any state. Highly recommended plans vary by year, but Utah, Nevada, and New York seem to always be at or near the top of the lists. The asset protection of HSAs, ESAs, and 529 accounts varies by state.

ABLE accounts are another tax-advantaged account available to the disabled. Think of an ABLE account as a 529 that can be used by your disabled child for their living expenses. The contribution limit is a little different in that it is $15,000 (2021) per beneficiary, no matter how many people open accounts or contribute to them. There is a 10% penalty on using the account for a non-allowed expense, but the definition of allowed expense is so broad I cannot imagine that penalty ever being enforced on something paid for in good faith. A few states do offer state tax deductions for contributions. Not every state offers an ABLE account yet, but they are becoming more popular so if this is a need for you, research the option in your state. You can learn more about ABLE accounts at *www.whitecoatinvestor.com/able-a-tax-protected-investing-account-for-your-special-child/*.

Understanding the basics of the tax code is a critical aspect of becoming financially literate. When you understand how taxes work, you can minimize the amount you pay by using the tax law to your advantage to reach your financial goals. For most doctors, retirement and other tax-protected plans are a key part of minimizing taxes. While tax evasion is illegal, tax avoidance (where you use legal methods to decrease your tax burden) is simply smart. You need to pay every dollar you owe, but you do not have to leave a tip.

MAIN IDEAS

- Your marginal tax rate is the rate at which your next dollar is taxed.

- Your effective tax rate is the taxes you pay divided by your income, and is a much better representation of your tax burden.

- The US Federal Income Tax is progressive, meaning you pay a higher percentage of your income as you make more money.

- Tax credits are more valuable than tax deductions.

- Tax rates on investments can be much lower than tax rates on earned income.

- The largest tax breaks available to most physicians are their retirement accounts.

- Maxing out your retirement accounts protects your money from taxes and creditors.

- Many physicians can use more than one 401(k), a health savings account, and a personal and spousal Backdoor Roth IRA.

ADDITIONAL RESOURCES

- **Resource:** Recommended Tax Strategists
  www.whitecoatinvestor.com/tax-strategists/

- **Blog Post:** Doctors Don't Pay 50% of Their Income in Taxes
  www.whitecoatinvestor.com/doctors-dont-pay-50-of-their-income-in-taxes/

- **Resource:** "I Want to Lower My Taxes" Is a Stupid Goal
  www.whitecoatinvestor.com/i-want-to-lower-my-taxes-is-a-stupid-goal/

- **Resource:** Tax-Deferred Retirement Accounts: A Gift from the Government
  www.whitecoatinvestor.com/tax-deferred-retirement-accounts-a-gift-from-the-government/

- **Resource:** Multiple 401(k) Rules
  www.whitecoatinvestor.com/multiple-401k-rules/

- **Resource:** Backdoor Roth IRA Tutorial
  www.whitecoatinvestor.com/backdoor-roth-ira-tutorial/

- **Resource:** The Stealth IRA
  www.whitecoatinvestor.com/retirement-accounts/the-stealth-ira/

- **Resource:** The 529 Account: A Tax Break for the Rich
  www.whitecoatinvestor.com/tax-break-for-the-rich-the-529-account-back-to-basics-series/

- **Resource:** ABLE: A Tax-Protected Investing Account for Your Special Child
  www.whitecoatinvestor.com/able-a-tax-protected-investing-account-for-your-special-child/

- **Resource:** 3 Ways Your 401(k) Lowers Your Tax Bill
  www.whitecoatinvestor.com/3-ways-your-401k-lowers-your-tax-bill/

CHAPTER TWENTY-ONE

FINANCIAL HISTORY

(FINANCIAL LITERACY 103)

Another important aspect of becoming financially literate is to have some sense of the history of financial instruments and markets. When you understand what has happened in the past, you will not be surprised to see it occur again in the present.[50] As I said earlier, while history does not necessarily repeat, it often rhymes.[51] Experienced investors, knowledgeable about past market history, do not panic in a market downturn. They say, "I have seen this movie before, and I know how it ends." This allows them to behave rationally when everyone else seems to be losing their heads.

One of the most devastating financial catastrophes for an investor is to repeatedly buy high and sell low. Just doing this once late in your career can mean working years longer than you would otherwise prefer. Yet our emotional, non-logical human brains are literally designed to do this. Knowing history will make you more patient and philosophical about enduring investment losses when they inevitably occur.

ANCIENT FINANCIAL HISTORY

In this chapter, we will perform a (very brief) review of economic history. Even ancient economic events provide useful lessons to be learned. For example, Hammurabi set up one of the first written legal systems in Babylon before his death in 1750 B.C. One section of the code defined interest rates:

"If a merchant has given corn on loan, he may take
100 SILA of corn as interest on 1 GUR; if he has
given silver on loan, he may take ⅙ shekel 6 grains
as interest on 1 shekel of silver."[52]

Essentially, this set interest rates at 20% on loans.[53]

3,000 years ago, the Talmud provided asset allocation advice to the Jewish people:

"Let every man divide his money into three parts,
and invest a third in land, a third in business and a
third let him keep by him in reserve."[54]

This passage essentially prescribes an asset allocation of ⅓ real estate, ⅓ stocks, and ⅓ cash or gold. (Jewish people did not charge or pay interest on loans to each other, so there were few bonds to invest in.)

The Knights Templar functioned as the original Western Union in many ways and invented many of the principles of accounting and banking still in use today. After the first crusade in 1099, many pilgrims would go to the "Holy Land," requiring many months worth of food, transport, and accommodation, but could not carry cash lest they become a target for robbers. The Knights Templar allowed a pilgrim to deposit money in London and withdraw it in Jerusalem months later while carrying nothing more than a letter of credit. While the Chinese government had a similar system of "flying money" run by the government centuries before the Knights, the Knights Templar were essentially the first private bank. The Knights also brokered deals and functioned as high-end pawnbrokers, once keeping the English Crown Jewels as security on a loan. For over 200 years, they were the financial system in Europe.

MODERN FINANCIAL HISTORY

Our modern banking system arose in Italy in the 1500s, which essentially created a currency that was not controlled by the kings of Europe. They performed currency exchange and offered lines of credit, settling up with each other every few months. For the first time, debt was being purchased and sold. One of Leonardo da Vinci's many contributions to our world was explaining and popularizing the use of double-entry bookkeeping, which is still used today in accounting and business. Fra Luca Pacioli, the father of accounting, wrote the book, and da Vinci did the illustrations!

The funding of voyages of exploration and international trade (unfortunately primarily of slaves) provided substantial difficulties in determining profits. The rulers of countries required a license in exchange for 20% of profits, but there were often no profits in those early centuries. The costs of providing ships and crews likely to mutiny and desert were not insubstantial and "cargo" could be surprisingly fragile to European diseases. Cutthroat competition between the various enterprises often resulted in armed conflict.

The first significant corporations also began to appear in Holland and England. Perhaps the best known of the early corporations was the English East India Company. These corporations were granted trade monopolies and in the early 1700s the East India Company was providing its investors annual returns of 150%! Naturally, it then went public. With the rise of Adam Smith inspired laissez-faire economic principles, by the early 1800s corporations in England were no longer government or guild associated. Laws were also passed in England, Germany, and the United States throughout the 19th century that shielded owners of corporations from liability.

A buttonwood tree on Wall Street in Manhattan was the origin of the New York Stock Exchange in the late 1700s, but the world's first significant stock exchange was in a roofless courtyard in Amsterdam in 1611. Stock exchanges allow owners of various corporations to buy and sell their shares and provide an opportunity for private companies to raise money by selling shares.

MANIAS (BUBBLES)

No financial history, no matter how brief, would be complete without at least some discussion of manias. Periodically throughout history, asset prices seem to rapidly rise in what is often called a financial mania or a speculative bubble, only to subsequently crash. Humans seem hard-wired to let their fear of missing out cause them to irrationally purchase assets at highly inflated prices in hopes of selling them to another speculator at an even higher price.

Perhaps the most famous of these manias is the Dutch Tulip Mania of the early 1600s. While this mania and its subsequent crash had no significant economic effect on the Netherlands, it demonstrated a hitherto unknown phenomenon that has been repeated periodically over the centuries since. While it seems difficult to believe now, certain rare tulip bulbs became incredibly valuable for a few short years. The tulip was introduced to Europe in the mid-1500s from the Ottoman Empire and by the 1600s was quite a status symbol in the Netherlands. Tulips flower for one week in April and May and then can be uprooted, sold, and replanted all summer during their dormant phase. A futures market (where you bought a contract in the spring to buy the bulb at the end of the summer) developed and short-selling, an important bubble control mechanism that provides downward pressure on prices, was outlawed.

At the peak of the bubble in February 1637, the most expensive tulips were trading at more than 10 times the annual income of a skilled laborer and one was once exchanged for 12 acres of land. Eventually, something that cannot continue forever must stop, and stop it did, when no buyers showed up at the tulip bulb auction on the 5th of February, 1637 (perhaps due to an outbreak of Bubonic Plague) and the prices dramatically collapsed.

Another famous bubble occurred in Britain. Second only to the East India Company, the South Seas Company also endured a speculative bubble, which caused investor Isaac Newton to exclaim "I can calculate the movement of the stars, but not the madness of men."[55] The company eventually became quite involved in the slave trade between Africa and the Spanish American colonies, but just nine years after its founding, the price of the stock went up from 100 pounds sterling to 1,000 pounds sterling in a single year. This attracted a great deal of attention to its shares among all classes of society, and to stocks in general. Another company advertised its shares as "a company for carrying out an undertaking of great advantage, but nobody to know what it is." Near the peak, the South Seas Company actually lent investors money to use to buy its own shares! The price collapsed back to 100 pounds sterling in August of 1720, triggering numerous bankruptcies and increased selling. An investigation ensued, massive corruption was found, the company's directors were sacked and stripped of, on average, 82% of their wealth, and the company stock was divided between the Bank of England and the East India Company. Robert Walpole, the First Lord of the Treasury, was credited with saving the British financial system and the government from total disgrace.

At about the same time as the South Seas Bubble, there was a similar event in France known as the Mississippi Company Bubble. This company was founded in 1684 and granted a trade monopoly with the French colonies in North America and the West Indies. John Law exaggerated the wealth of Louisiana after his visit and due to very effective marketing, investors became very excited about the company's prospects. Share prices rapidly climbed and the company actually combined with the Royal Bank, paying out dividends in banknotes. Eventually, the bank admitted it did not have enough gold and silver coins to cover all of the banknotes and when people tried to turn in the notes for actual coins, the bubble burst as the bank refused to redeem the notes. In essence, this was less a speculative event and more of a currency blunder (Law took the currency off of the gold standard and put it on the Mississippi Company share price standard), but given that it occurred in the same year as the British South Seas Company Bubble, they tend to be lumped together.

From 1790 to 1810 in England there was another speculative event, usually referred to as the Canal Mania. Canals dramatically reduced the cost of shipping goods, and thus could make great profit. While records are scant, over this time period, there were at least three speculative bubbles. The shares of the Grand Junction Canal were issued in 1790 at 100 pounds sterling and increased to 472 pounds sterling before the canal was even approved by the government, much less actually started! By 1795, they were back to the par value of 100. The London Stock Exchange was established in 1801, so the second two bubbles, while not quite as dramatic, were more inviting to investors.

The 1800s saw several impressively bad economic periods in the United States, beginning in 1819, 1837, 1857, 1873, and 1893. The first of these, referred to either as The Panic of 1819 or The First Great Depression, occurred as a result of events that occurred in Europe in the aftermath of the Napoleonic Wars. It certainly included a speculative or bubble aspect. Great Britain was producing more goods than Continental Europe could absorb, so they unloaded them at low prices in the US. Meanwhile, the US found a new market in Europe for foodstuffs, tobacco, and cotton, especially after The Year without a Summer after the eruption of Mount Tambor and the resulting agricultural failures. This increase in demand for US agricultural products resulted in a speculative land boom in the Southern and Western United States. It was fueled by loans from a relatively unregulated and precious-metals-poor banking system. When Europe recovered, the price of agricultural goods dropped and land prices collapsed. Banks, unable to redeem their own notes with gold and silver, foreclosed on properties, decreasing their value by 50–75%. The price of cotton dropped 25% in one day, triggering a recession. There was plenty of blame to go around, but most of it fell on the brand-new Second Bank of the United States and its conservative fiscal policies.

We now turn our attention back to the United Kingdom. Just as canals made it easier, cheaper, and faster to ship goods, so did a new technology—railroads. During the 1840s, a speculative event in railway stocks occurred, peaking in 1846. As usual, as the price of stock increased, investors invested more and more (including with borrowed money) and the price increased further. 272 Acts of Parliament establishing railroads were passed in 1846 at the peak, although ⅓ of authorized railways were never built. There were a lot of contributing factors to the bubble. In 1825, the Bubble Act (passed after the South Seas Bubble in 1720) was repealed, allowing for an enlarging middle class to invest.

Newspapers (new at the time) spread the word rapidly, and the stock market made it easy to buy and sell shares. In fact, you could buy shares with just a 10% down payment, allowing the company to call the rest of your purchase at any time. Unfortunately, this resulted in people using their entire savings to buy 10 times as many shares as they should have. Many of them were completely wiped out, but at least there was a nice side effect of this bubble—Britain was left with thousands of miles of railways, over half of what currently exists. Interestingly, the United States had its own little railway boom after the Civil War, especially in the 1880s, with a bust in 1894 when ¼ of railroad companies went bankrupt. Speculation in railroad stocks also contributed to the Panics of 1857 and 1873, discussed below.

The Panic of 1837 (also sometimes known as The First Great Depression) also had a speculative element. Its causes were surprisingly similar to those of 1819—speculative lending in Western states with a resulting land price bubble and a drop in the price of cotton. As lending practices tightened in response, the banks again refused to redeem their own notes for gold and silver, triggering a seven-year period of falling wages, falling profits, falling prices, and rising unemployment, which was as high as 25% at the peak. In essence, the British were speculating in American enterprises and land. In 1836, to curb speculation, a law (Specie Circular) was passed that required Western lands to be purchased only with gold and silver, and both land and commodity prices dropped dramatically. There was a massive loss of confidence and runs on banks were common. 343 of the 850 banks in the United States failed. Numerous states defaulted on their bonds, leaving

British investors in the lurch and the United States even withdrew from international money markets for a while. This prolonged economic downturn and deflationary period really did not improve until the Gold Rush of the late 1840s.

The economic boom-bust periods of the 1800s continued, with the next bust in 1857. Many consider The Panic of 1857 to be the first worldwide economic crisis. In many ways, it was triggered by the Dred Scott Supreme Court decision, where Dred Scott sued for his freedom but was denied because of the color of his skin. The Missouri Compromise was declared unconstitutional and this uncertainty in the development of the West led to the end of a speculative rise in railroad stocks. The banks holding many shares of the stocks were then put under pressure. The price of grain also fell, putting more pressure on banks as farmers could not make their mortgage payments. This recession was much shorter than in 1837 and primarily affected the North.

The Panic of 1873 was called The Great Depression, at least up until 1929! Another worldwide depression, it was known in Britain as The Long Depression and contributed significantly to the decline of the British Empire. As usual, the run-up involved a time of great prosperity and increasing speculation and lax lending policies. The immediate trigger was a fall in silver prices (mostly mined in the US) when Germany stopped minting silver thalers. The US went to a de facto gold standard. The domestic money supply decreased, interest rates went up, and the heavily indebted went into crisis mode. Banks, insurance companies, railroads, and other businesses (18,000 total) failed. Railroad and building construction ceased, factories were closed, wages were cut, real estate values fell, and profits disappeared. The stock exchange was even closed for 10 days. In many ways, this economic downturn was the cause of the failure of Reconstruction, the consequences of which are still being felt in 2020. The depression was over by 1879, but lingering tensions between labor and capital continued onward after the strikes, protests, and civil unrest that occurred during the depression. Unemployment peaked at just over 8%.

The Panic of 1893 was triggered by speculation by Europeans in Argentina, South Africa and Australia. When these collapsed, investors demanded metal coins from US banks. The failure of the Reading Railroad (of Monopoly fame) was one of the first signs of trouble in the US and the bank runs started as people lost confidence and credit collapsed, triggering a four-year depression. Over 15,000 companies, including 500 banks, failed.

Unemployment peaked as high as 43% in Michigan and when the loss of income was combined with the loss of their life savings due to the bank failures, the middle class was largely wiped out and had to walk away from their homes due to not being able to meet their mortgage obligations. Hunger and desperation were widespread. As usual, the economy gradually recovered as confidence improved.

The 1920s saw a speculative event in Florida real estate. While Florida has had several real estate bubbles, this was the first and most impressive. It was the usual story: out of state speculators, easy credit, and rapidly rising prices creating a vicious cycle. A new railroad to Florida combined with the difficulty in traveling to Europe due to World War I and the general prosperity in the US to set the stage. At its peak, the same property was being sold at auction as often as 10 times a day. Prices quadrupled in 1925. One property bought for $1,700 later sold for $300,000. By 1926, things were fizzling out. Two hurricanes and the 1929 stock market crash finished it off. Florida was not the only place to see real estate prices fall after the 1920s. In 1940, Manhattan real estate was selling for just 41% of its 1920 price.

The "Roaring 20s" (1925–1929) were a time of prosperity, increasing consumer debt, and increasing economic speculation, particularly in the stock market. Increasing numbers of investors were becoming rich, at least on paper. Joe Kennedy (father of JFK) famously described the scene:

> "Taxi drivers told you what to buy. The shoeshine boy could give you a summary of the day's financial news as he worked with rag and polish. An old beggar who regularly patrolled the street in front of my office now gave me tips and, I suppose, spent the money I and others gave him in the market. My cook had a brokerage account and followed the ticker closely. Her paper profits were quickly blown away in the gale of 1929."[56]

The stock market collapse in 1929 was just the beginning. Manufacturing ground to a halt. Crop prices fell by 60%, despite a massive drought which caused 10% of farms to change hands. Unemployment soared. Over 9,000 banks failed. The market crashed 90%, recovered somewhat, then crashed again, scaring an entire generation into investing only in bonds the rest of their lives. Unemployment remained high until World War II; it was still

15% in 1940. It seems with The Great Depression, we finally learned our lesson and passed a number of important regulatory laws to prevent it from happening again.

One of the most important was the Banking Act of 1933. This Act established the Federal Deposit Insurance Corporation (FDIC), a very important aspect of our banking system that solved many of the issues that caused the repeated panics from 1819 to 1929. Now if a bank failed, the federal government stepped in and made the depositors whole. All of a sudden, there was no more need to start a run on the bank. You just had to wait a little bit for the FDIC to come in and give you your money back. Currently, up to $250,000 per depositor per bank is insured. (In 1970, a similar insurance fund was established for credit unions.) Franklin Delano Roosevelt, our longest-serving president, was elected in 1933. Society was dramatically transformed by a number of pieces of legislation passed while he was president. One of the most significant was the establishment of Social Security. Prior to this time, the only option for those who found themselves old or disabled without much savings was to rely on family or charity. Other important pieces of financial legislation passed as a result of the Great Depression include:

- The Securities Act of 1933
- The Securities Exchange Act of 1934
- The Trust Indenture Act of 1939
- The Investment Company Act of 1940
- The Investment Advisers Act of 1940

All of these important pieces of legislation are still in effect and determine how stock exchanges, mutual funds, advisors, and others act today.

The Poseidon Bubble was a speculative stock market bubble in Australian mining stocks in 1969 and 1970. Nickel was in high demand at the time and a company called Poseidon Nickel found a big nickel deposit in September 1969. The shares went from 80 cents to $280 per share. It quickly spread to other mining stocks and the mining index went up 44% in two months. It all came crashing down in early 1970. The price of nickel soon fell, compounding issues for Poseidon which went into bankruptcy by 1974.

The Nifty Fifty was a set of 50 "blue-chip" stocks in the US that were considered "can't lose" investments in the late 1960s and early 1970s. They often traded at up to 50 times earnings due to solid earnings growth. They outperformed until the 1973–1974 stock market crash, then underperformed for years (except Wal-Mart). Most eventually did okay as companies, but it was a good example of the dangers of overpaying for growth stocks that reminds many investors of the rise of the FAANG stocks (see below) in the late 2010s.

Silver Thursday refers to an attempt to "corner the silver market" in 1979–1980 by the Hunt brothers. These wealthy brothers had purchased as much as ⅓ of the silver in the world at one point. The price of silver had risen from $6 an ounce to almost $50 an ounce. The silver exchanges changed their rules on the Hunt brothers, limiting the amount of leverage they were allowed to use. They were unable to meet their obligations and the price collapsed 50% over just four days. This was the first of the speculative bubbles that affected my life. While I was only four years old on Silver Thursday, I have a recollection of my parents owning a bucket of silver coins that were stored in my closet as a child when I was about that age. I suspect they took a pretty good haircut on them!

In the 1980s, Japan was all the rage. The value of shares of Japanese companies as well as Japanese real estate soared on a strong Yen. One look at a long-term graph of the Japanese stock market index demonstrates the problem well. Between 1980 and the peak at the end of 1989, the Nikkei 225 Index rose from 6,000 to almost 40,000, before crashing to about 14,000 over the course of a year. The remarkable thing is that as I pen this chapter 30 years later, the Nikkei 225 is still only at 23,000. If you overpay enough for something, you may never get back to even.

1997 brought the Asian Financial Crisis, which affected many Southeast Asian countries, but none more severely than Thailand. These countries had their currencies pegged to the US dollar, which had been strengthening over the previous few years. Thailand had been a darling for investors, offering high-interest rates and an average GDP growth rate of 9% over the previous decade. The crisis started when Thailand ran out of foreign currency to support its pegged currency and had to devalue it. Panic quickly spread to other countries. Currency and stock market values fell (75% in Thailand). Even the US stock market was affected, although not as severely. Developed market investors certainly became much more careful about lending money to developing countries. This contributed to the famous meltdown of Long

Term Capital Management, a hedge fund counting two Noble laureates on its staff, the next year when Russia defaulted on its sovereign debt. At one point, this highly leveraged fund had just $400 million in equity and over $100 billion in debt. It was bailed out by the US Federal Reserve to prevent collapse of the entire financial system.

The late 1990s were a time of significant speculation. One of the more interesting of these were small stuffed animals called Beanie Babies. By 1995, they became an internet sensation. People began to collect them not only as toys, but as a financial investment. The company deliberately made certain Beanie Babies scarce, retiring certain models before coming out with new ones, maintaining a scarcity due to low supply and high demand. Authorities even assisted by cracking down hard on counterfeiters. These toys were initially sold at $5, but sold at the peak in 1999 for as much as $13,000 each. They were fought over in divorce court. They were stolen. They were smuggled. This speculative bubble even led to at least one murder of a security guard. Something that cannot continue forever eventually does not, and when Ty, Inc. announced the retirement of a few models and their value did not increase dramatically for the first time, a switch flipped. Prices collapsed 90–99% almost overnight, and with it a significant portion of a few investors' college and retirement funds.

The most impressive speculative event of the late 1990s was the Dot. com Bubble. As the 1990s went on, more and more people in the US and across the globe started using the internet. It was easy to see that it would transform the way we live and do business. Just like other new technologies (canals, railroads, airlines), investors would fund almost any project. Just adding ".com" to the end of a company's name increased its price by 74%. (Interestingly enough, just a few years after the bubble burst, removing ".com" from a company name also increased its price by 64%.) The Nasdaq stock exchange was where most of these new, internet-centric companies were listed. Its index rose 400% between 1995 and 2000. It finally peaked in March 2000 with a price to earnings ratio of 200.

By that point, investors were buying shares in internet companies at any valuation. Many of these companies had no significant assets or even revenue, much less earnings. People were quitting their jobs left and right to spend their time day trading stocks. Doctors were trading stocks online between patients. At the same time, there was a bit of a bubble in Telecom companies. They were busy putting in fiber optic cable, switches, and networks that would be needed in the new "Information Age." Otherwise sensible investing books published in the late 1990s recommended investors allocate 5% of their portfolio to technology stocks and another 5% to telecom stocks. It all came crashing down over a period of about a month in 2000, and stock prices continued spiraling downward for two more years. At the bottom in 2002, the Nasdaq had lost 78% of its value and many ".com" companies were completely out of business. Others, such as Cisco, took major hits. Even the winners of the internet boom such as eBay and Amazon had large drops in value prior to recovering. While investors did not seem to swear off stocks, many certainly swore off day trading! Many parallels can be seen to the rise of day trading again in 2020 at the hands of populist brokerage firms such as Robinhood and Webull.

In response to the stock market crash and economic downturn associated with the dot.com crash, interest rates were lowered dramatically. They were lowered so much that most of my medical school classmates refinanced their student loans at less than 1% when we graduated in 2003. This easy money fueled the next speculative event, the US housing bubble. In many states, home prices soared. Many of my residency classmates had their home prices in Tucson double from 2003 to 2006 when we graduated. Lending standards were more and more relaxed as the lenders found they could sell the resulting debt off to investors. Even relatively risky subprime loans became attractive to investors once they were packaged up with other similarly risky loans. It spread to other countries as well. Home flipping became so popular that numerous TV shows popped up showing how to do it. Many homeowners refinanced or took out home equity lines of credit, and used the proceeds to purchase consumer items or fund living expenses. Real estate investing was all the rage.

Eventually, the ratio of home price to income for homeowners and the ratio of home price to rent for investors became unsustainable and in 2005–2007 (depending on location) prices started to collapse. In some areas, this decline in pricing continued until 2012. The median home price fell 6% from 2006 to 2007, but even that decline reflected the sticky pricing of such an illiquid asset. Fewer and fewer homes were being sold at all, and those who had bought with risky interest-only, zero-down mortgages they could not afford found themselves mailing their keys into their lenders. In 2007, the subprime mortgage market collapsed, with no fewer than 25 federally insured lenders going out of business.

By Fall 2008, large national banks (considered too big to fail) required government bailouts, the stock market crashed almost 50%, and a recession began. Median housing prices only fell 22% nationwide, but in some areas of the country (such as Las Vegas), prices fell as much as 75%. Those who had bought with little down found themselves underwater, meaning they owed more than the property was worth. Even those who had put down a real down payment and had been in their home for years found themselves underwater, especially if they had been using their home equity as an ATM. On an inflation-adjusted basis, the median housing price did not recover until 2019. Las Vegas housing still has not returned to its peak when this chapter was written in 2020.

As a student of financial history, I thought I would never be the witness of a true mania like the Dutch Tulip Bulb Mania. However, I was wrong. The first decentralized cryptocurrency, Bitcoin, popped up in 2009. Since then over 6,000 other cryptocurrencies or coins have been created. Cryptocurrencies, and particularly Bitcoin, became more and more popular as the years went on. While it was rarely used as a currency, and was frankly far too volatile to be a stable store of value, it served well as a speculative instrument. In 2011, you could buy a Bitcoin for just $0.30. By 2012, a Bitcoin was worth $5.12. In 2013, the price went from $13.30 to $770 per Bitcoin and people really started paying attention, just in time for an 87% crash in value.

That certainly cooled off interest among investors, but by 2016, the value had recovered completely, which set the stage for a truly remarkable 2017. By mid-summer, prices had risen from $998 to $2,748 and everybody knew about it. There were articles in the paper every day and the nurses in the ER were dreaming of becoming Bitcoin millionaires. As Fall turned into Winter, it was obvious to any student of financial history that this was a classic mania. The price eventually peaked on December 17th at $19,783.06. By December 22nd, it was back down to $15,075. By April 2018, it was under $7,000 per Bitcoin. By the time a year had passed from the peak, Bitcoins were trading for $3,183, a decline of 84%. At the end of 2020 as this book is being edited, Bitcoin is climbing rapidly and has surpassed its former peak. The most impressive thing about the 2017 Bitcoin Mania was just how quickly it happened. From mid-November to mid-December 2017, the price of Bitcoin rose 154% in value from $7,777 to $19,783, and that was after the price had already increased seven-fold in the first 11 months of the year!

As this book is being written, we are in the midst of the rise of the FAANG stocks (Facebook, Apple, Amazon, Netflix, and Google). These internet-based companies have been darlings for individual and institutional investors alike for the last few years. Tesla could also be easily added to the list. In December 2020, it has a trailing P/E ratio of nearly 100 when the average among other automotive manufacturers is about 29. Even its founder and CEO, Elon Musk, says the value is "too high." Only time will tell how this particular episode will turn out.

SIGNS OF A BUBBLE

I know I have spent a lot of space talking about the various financial manias and speculative events in history, but being forewarned is being forearmed. These will not be the last manias, and I want you to be able to recognize future manias when they occur. Author, physician, and financial advisor William Bernstein says there are four signs of a bubble, and when you see all four of them, you should steer clear![57]

1. Everybody starts talking about the bubble asset. The classic example is shoeshine boys giving stock tips in 1929, but I have seen this occur also with Beanie Babies, dot.com stocks, houses, and Bitcoin. If people who are not normally investors are talking about and investing in an asset class, it might be time to get out!

2. People begin quitting their jobs to day trade, become a mortgage broker, or otherwise get involved in the bubble industry.

3. When someone exhibits skepticism about the prospects for the bubble asset, people do not just disagree with them, but they do so vehemently and tell them they are an idiot for not understanding things.

4. When you start to see extreme predictions. In 1999, there was a book published that was called *Dow $36,000*.[58] The day Bitcoin peaked in December 2017, CNBC had an analyst on TV predicting that it would soon be worth $300,000–$400,000, and felt that was a "conservative call."[59]

Keep these four signs in mind as you move throughout your investing career. Stay rational, stay diversified, and enjoy the show from the sidelines. Emotion is not your friend in investing and one of the most difficult things for a long-term investor is to keep your head when everyone else is losing theirs. I cannot overemphasize the fact that the investor, and his or her temperament, matter far more than the actual investments used.

SHALLOW RISK VERSUS DEEP RISK

While we are talking about Bernstein, we should discuss the true risks that your portfolio faces. Risk is often measured using standard deviation, a measure of volatility. Obviously, if your portfolio declines by 50% right when you need that money, it is going to cause you some real-life financial issues. However, for a long-term rational investor, mere volatility is not necessarily something to be feared. So what if it takes three, four, or even 10 years for your investment to provide a solid return if you do not need that money for decades? Bernstein calls volatility a "shallow risk," something for investing neophytes to fear, but not something "investing adults" should fear.[60] An "investing adult," i.e. a rational, knowledgeable investor, should fear permanent loss of capital. If you have a sensible, diversified portfolio, that permanent loss really only occurs through four mechanisms—inflation, deflation, confiscation, and devastation. These "four horsemen" of true risk have reared their heads at various times in history and it is worth knowing about these incidents.

The most common "deep risk" is inflation, and specifically hyperinflation. The US Federal Reserve targets an inflation rate of about 2%. A little inflation is thought by economists to be a good thing that helps economies to grow. However, they are unanimous that out of control inflation is a bad thing. In 1980, inflation peaked at nearly 15%. At those rates, both consumer and investor behavior are severely affected, and that has dire effects on an economy. Over the course of a decade, a 15% inflation rate can turn $100 into just $20. However, even that is not considered "hyper" inflation. For that, we have to turn to other countries.

After World War I, Germany was forced to make reparation payments in currency other than German currency. This resulted in German currency having an inflation rate of more than 30,000% per month!

In Hungary after World War II, inflation reached 200%. Per day. By 1946, you could buy every bit of currency in Hungary with ⅒oth of one US penny.

More recently, inflation spiraled out of control in Zimbabwe in the late 2000s, reaching rates of 79 billion percent per month. They had to print $200 million notes and the price of bread reached $35 million. Imagine having to take a wheelbarrow of cash to the store in order to buy whatever they have there since almost anything will be more valuable than the banknotes!

Obviously, this type of inflation will devastate an economy and many investments. Long-term nominal bonds in particular are at risk of inflation.

The second deep risk is deflation, which is a prolonged period of economic contraction. One of the best examples is The Great Depression. Unemployment soars, property and company values fall, and although prices are attractive, nobody actually has any money to buy anything. Since everything falls in value, the mere fall in value is not as bad as the economic consequences that typically accompany it: a severe and prolonged decrease in economic activity.

The third deep risk, confiscation, is no small risk either. Just ask an investor in 1918 Russia who saw the new communist government take everything he had. Confiscation can happen directly, or indirectly via high taxation or even deliberately high inflation. While the Russian example is at one extreme, a Wikipedia article titled "List of Nationalizations by Country"[61] lists hundreds of examples ranging from the nationalization of airline security companies in the US after 9/11 (heard of TSA?) to the 2010 seizure of US oil company assets and French grocery stores by Venezuela.

Finally, devastation is the fourth deep risk. Imagine owning a handful of successful businesses in 1945 Hiroshima. Or perhaps stock in a real estate company in 1871 Chicago, where over 3 square miles of the city was destroyed by fire. Need a more modern example? Take a look at Aleppo during the recent (ongoing?) Syrian Civil War. While war is perhaps the most common cause of devastation, natural disasters are frequent contributors. In fact, the COVID-19 pandemic is one form of economic devastation that few saw coming. While it is not clear how much of a long-term economic impact this will have on the world at the time of writing this chapter, it has absolutely devastated many parts of the world economy from conventions to theaters to airlines.

SETTING EXPECTATIONS

Understanding financial history helps you to understand the real risks you face in your investing career. It can also help you to weather economic storms in real-time when you understand just how severe economic events in the past have been. It is much easier to adopt a philosophical attitude of "This too shall pass" when you realize how many times in history people have overcome severe economic disruption. Consider the frequency of stock market corrections (an overall drop of 10% in value of the stock market) and bear markets (an overall drop of 20% in value of the stock market). If you look at stock market data you will see that these are relatively frequent events. From 1980 to 2020 (40 years), there have been 38 corrections. Essentially, these occur about once a year on average. So if you are an investor for 30 years during your career and 30 years during your retirement, you should expect to have to endure about 60 corrections. It should not be a surprise to run into one. It is an expected event, and you should have a plan for what to do when it does occur (refuse to sell low, rebalance your investments, and perhaps buy even more of the beaten-up asset classes at an attractive price). Corrections have averaged a 15.6% decline over that time period and recoveries typically take four months. About one out of four times that correction became a bear market.

Since 1927, there have been about 17 bear markets. So on average, you should expect one about every five years. Sometimes these are very brief (on October 22, 1987 the stock market dropped 22.6% in one day, but had recovered by the end of the year) and sometimes they last for years. On average, a bear market takes 627 days to go from the market high to market low, and takes about four years total to make a full recovery. Again, if you expect to be an investor for 60 years, you should expect to have to pass through about 12 of these. It is an expected event.

It can also be useful to look at the performance of various asset classes historically. In 1999, Jay Koepfer created the first Callan Periodic Table of Investment Returns. This table, updated each year, demonstrates how the various types of stocks and bonds have performed against each other in any given year. You can see the table at *www.callan.com/periodic-table/*. You do not have to stare at the table for long to realize that every investment has its day in the sun and that chasing performance is likely a fool's errand. For example, Emerging Market stocks were the best asset class on the chart in 2003, 2005, 2007, 2009, and 2017, but the worst asset class on the chart in 2008, 2011, 2015, and 2018. Real estate outperformed US stocks in 11 of the last 20 years. Likewise, small stocks outperformed large stocks 11 out of 20 years. The take-away message is printed right on the chart these days:

> "The Callan Periodic Table of Investment Returns conveys the strong case for diversification across asset classes (stocks versus bonds), capitalizations (large versus small), and equity markets (U.S.

versus global ex-U.S.). The Table highlights the uncertainty inherent in all capital markets. Rankings change every year. Also noteworthy is the difference between absolute and relative performance, as returns for the top-performing asset class span a wide range over the past 20 years."[62]

The message you should take is explained well by the late Jack Bogle, founder of Vanguard. He called it "reversion to the mean" and described it as a "kind of law of gravity in the stock market through which returns mysteriously seem to be drawn to norms of one kind or another over time."[63] In his writing, he compared value stocks to growth stocks, low-priced stocks to high-priced stocks, small stocks to large stocks, and US stocks to international stocks. In each case, he demonstrated that over long periods of time, returns were similar, even though there were periods of time in which one would outperform the other.

It is also useful for an investor to understand historical returns of various investments. While there is no guarantee that future returns will be the same as past returns, the range of historical returns does provide an investor with a reasonable idea of what is possible.

The average annualized return of the US stock market from 1871 to present, including dividends, is 9.19% per year (7% after inflation). The return has been positive in 2 out of every 3 calendar years. However, with a standard deviation of over 18%, the return is rarely anywhere near 9%. It is usually either much more or much less. In fact, over the last 150 years, the return has been over 20% 45 times![64] So you should not be surprised to earn 25% or 30% on your stocks in a given year, it happens all the time. You also should not be surprised to take a loss on those same stocks the next year, since that happens about as often as the really high return years.

What about bonds? According to Vanguard, from 1926 to 2018, a 100% bond portfolio had an annualized return of 5.3%, significantly lower than stocks. In its best year (1982) this portfolio had a return of 32.6% and in its worst year (1969) it had a loss of 8.1%. It lost money in 14 out of 93 years, about half as often as stocks. They also provide data for the "classic" 60/40 portfolio, comprised of 60% stocks and 40% bonds. Over that same time period, this portfolio had an annualized return of 8.6% and lost money in 22 out of 93 years. Both its best and worst year occurred in the Great Depression, 36.7% in 1933 and -26.6% in 1931.[65]

Long-term data can be pretty sparse for many types of investments, but one "alternative" investment whose long-term returns we know is gold. 800 years ago, an ounce of gold bought a nice man's suit. Today, an ounce of gold buys a nice man's suit. Gold generally keeps up with inflation, but does not necessarily beat it. Jeremy Siegel, in his book *Stocks for the Long Run*,[66] famously demonstrated that over the course of 196 years, $10,000 invested in stocks would grow to $5.6 billion, after inflation. That same $10,000 invested in bonds would grow to $8 million. While nowhere near $5.6 billion, it is still a good sum of money. What if you had invested that same $10,000 in gold? Well, you would now have $25,000 worth of gold.

It can also be helpful to understand what interest rates have been in the past. We opened this chapter with a discussion of the 20% interest rates in ancient Babylon. Throughout history, the more stable and prosperous a society, the lower its interest rates tended to be. As discussed above in the section on deep risks, the only interest rate that matters is the real, or after-inflation interest rate, but for the sake of convenience, I will be using nominal (non-inflation adjusted) rates below. In order to convert those to real rates, simply subtract the rate of inflation (which has averaged 2–4% per year over the last century).

Certain interest rates can be set by government entities, while others fluctuate in the markets. In the US, the Federal Reserve set an interest rate known as the Federal Funds Rate, the rate at which banks lend each other money overnight. Between 1954 and today, this rate has varied between 0.25% and 19%. Perhaps a better indicator of interest rates is the 10-year treasury rate. In 1960, this rate was about 4%. This rate climbed throughout the 70s as inflation reared its ugly head, peaking at 15.5% in 1981 and has generally been on a declining trend since that time. It passed back below 4% after the dot.com bust before rising.

Since the 2008 Global Financial Crisis, these yields have remained below 4% and have even been below 1% as they are at the time of this writing. Another useful interest rate is the rate of the 30-year mortgage. In 1971, this was just below 8% before rising to 16.6% in 1981. Since then, rates have gradually declined until the present, when a 30-year mortgage can be had for about 3%.[67] Predicting future interest rates can be just as difficult as predicting stock market returns, but it is helpful to know where we have been in the past. I occasionally hear someone worry about interest rates going up to 4% before they can lock in their mortgage and it makes me chuckle, remembering my first mortgage in 1999, which was 8%. The house I grew up in was purchased in 1979 with a double-digit interest rate.

Likewise, it can be helpful to understand what federal income tax rates have been in the past. While relatively few people ever find themselves in the top tax bracket, this bracket has ranged from 7% when the modern federal income tax was implemented to 91–92% in the 1950s before falling to 28% (Reagan era), 35% (George W. Bush era), and 37% (Trump era). Effective tax rates, even on the wealthy, have not been so extreme. While they also climbed between 1913 and the 1950s, throughout the 1950s the top 1% paid about 42% of their income in taxes. This number has fluctuated between 31% and 46% since.[68]

Historical Tax Rates

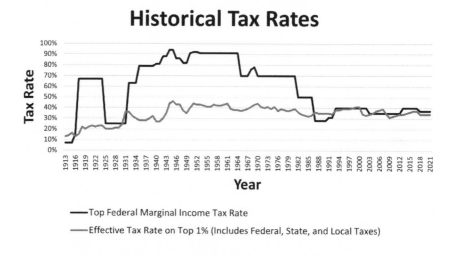

—Top Federal Marginal Income Tax Rate

⋯⋯Effective Tax Rate on Top 1% (Includes Federal, State, and Local Taxes)

What does that number look like for the rest of society? In 2016, 33% of tax returns had a negative effective tax rate. That is right, they actually received more back than they paid. Another 42% paid less than 10% in taxes. 22% paid 10–20% in taxes. Only about 2.5% of returns had an effective tax rate over 20%.

State income tax rates are highly variable, ranging from 0% in seven states (Alaska, Florida, Nevada, South Dakota, Texas, Wyoming, Washington) to 13.3% for the highest earners in California. Most states have a progressive income tax system, where higher earners pay a higher rate, but 11 states have a flat income tax system, where everybody pays the same rate. These flat rates are typically in the 4–5% range.

If you want to be successful at personal finance and investing, it is very helpful to understand financial history. If you know where we have been, you will have the proper perspective on current economic events. Perspective may be the most valuable of intellectual commodities. Perspective brings everything together and allows your brain and its skills to operate properly. You should continually assess and improve your perspective. It will allow you to make better decisions about earning, saving, investing, borrowing, spending, and giving.

MAIN IDEAS

- Understanding financial history allows you to put current economic and political events in the proper perspective.

- It is normal for markets to have severe fluctuations periodically.

- Occasionally, markets go stark raving mad and a bubble or mania forms. These are more easily recognized if you are familiar with past manias.

- The long-term investor is much more concerned about deep risk (risk of permanent loss) than shallow risk (temporary volatility).

- Most investments will have their day in the sun. Avoid performance chasing.

ADDITIONAL RESOURCES

- **Resource:** Callan Table of Periodic Returns
  www.callan.com/periodic-table/

- **Blog Post:** Understanding Market History Provides Perspective
  www.whitecoatinvestor.com/understanding-market-history-adds-perspective/

- **Blog Post:** Cryptocurrencies like Bitcoin Are Not Investments
  www.whitecoatinvestor.com/cryptocurrencies-like-bitcoin-are-not-investments/

- **Blog Post:** The Savings Rate
  www.whitecoatinvestor.com/investing/the-savings-rate/

CHAPTER TWENTY-TWO

NUMBERS YOU NEED TO KNOW

(FINANCIAL LITERACY 104)

So far in this financial literacy section of the book we have discussed investments, the tax code (including the special tax-protected investing accounts available to you), and a brief overview of financial history. Another important aspect of being financially literate is becoming adept with numbers. Do not worry, we are not going to be talking about trigonometry and calculus here. You learned all of the math you need to know to be financially savvy by the time you finished the fifth grade. Anything harder than that can be done using a financial calculator.

There are a handful of calculations worth doing periodically throughout your life. The first of these is the primary measure of wealth, net worth. Too many people think income is the proper measure of wealth. Popular culture and even the US government get this wrong. However, someone who makes $500,000 a year and spends $500,000 a year might have a high income, but will never become wealthy. Wealth is what you have left after you get done spending. As Morgan Housel famously said,

> "The truth is [that] people need to be told that if you spend money on things, you will end up with the things and not the money. When most people say they want to be a millionaire, what they really mean is "I want to spend a million dollars," which is literally the opposite of being a millionaire."[69]

NET WORTH

Truly, you become a millionaire by not spending a million dollars you could have spent. Net worth is simply everything you own minus everything you owe. Technically it includes not only your bank account, retirement accounts, the value of your practice, and other investments, but also the value of your home and everything in it from your automobiles to your jewelry to the items in your broom closet. Practically speaking, most people only include financial accounts, investments, and the value of their home since all of those smaller items are so hard to value accurately. Once you have added up all of your assets, you simply need to subtract all of your debts, also called liabilities. See what I mean about grade school math? This stuff is not that hard.

So subtract any mortgage you may have, practice-related debt, your student loans, your car loan, and the balances of your credit cards. Assets minus liabilities equals net worth. If you will calculate this each year, you will accurately track your progress toward wealth, and more importantly, your own financial goals. Granted, it will likely be a bit depressing to calculate this out during medical school, dental school, or residency since the total will likely be quite negative. Pour yourself a favorite beverage and do it anyway. It will later give you a real sense of accomplishment to know how far you have come. Using net worth as the measurement, the typical medical or dental school graduate is actually one of the poorest people in the world, typically with a net worth that ranges from -$100,000 to -$500,000.

It is not that income does not matter. It certainly does. It is the most important wealth-building tool that a typical doctor has. It is also pretty easy to calculate. In fact, you probably do not even have to do it on your own. Just look at your tax return from last year. On the 2019 1040, line 7b is the "Total Income" line. While it is not necessarily a perfect measurement, it is good enough for our purposes. This is the total of all of your salaries, business profits, interest, and investment dividends. To be even more accurate, you may wish to add in the money your employer pulled from your paychecks to place in your retirement accounts on your behalf, along with the provided employer match.

TAX RATES

There are two tax rates worth calculating as well. The first is your marginal tax rate. This is closely related to the sum of your federal and state tax brackets, but also includes some payroll taxes such as Social Security and Medicare taxes. The easiest way to calculate it is to use tax software. Once you have done your taxes for the year (or your accountant has) add another $100 to your income. How much did your tax bill go up? That is your marginal tax rate. If another $100 of income raised your taxes by $38, you have a marginal tax rate of 38%. 38% of every additional dollar you earn will go to the taxman.

The other important tax rate is your effective tax rate. This is easier to calculate. Again, pull out your tax return from last year. Look at your "Total Income" (line 7b on the 2019 1040) and your "Total Tax" (line 16 on the 2019 1040). If you divide your "Total Tax" by your "Total Income," that will tell you your effective tax rate. If you want to be completely accurate, subtract any tax credits you received (lines 18a-c) from your "Total Tax." Of course, you will need to also add any state income taxes you paid to your "Total Tax." A higher effective tax rate is not necessarily a bad thing, since it usually means you made more money and the instances where earning more money causes you to have less money after tax are very rare in the tax code.

SAVINGS RATE

Our next worthwhile calculation is your retirement savings rate. I think this is worth calculating once per year throughout your working career and I encourage doctors who have finished their training to aim for a rate of at least 20%. This is simply how much money you saved for retirement divided by how much money you earned (again, "Total Income" from your tax return). Be sure to include contributions to retirement accounts, including any employer match, in both the numerator and denominator of the equation. If you will save 20% of your gross income for retirement throughout your career, you will be able to maintain your standard of living during retirement. You will need to save more if you wish to retire early. Remember that 20% does not include paying off debt, saving up for a new car, or saving for college.

FINANCIAL CALCULATORS

Now that we have done the basic calculations, I wanted to introduce you to some more complex calculations. Do not worry, you will not have to do these yourself. You simply use a calculator or a spreadsheet. If you have any interest whatsoever in becoming wealthy during your life, I highly recommend you learn to use these simple tools. A typical spreadsheet like Microsoft Excel or Google Sheets will walk you through these calculations. While I am not going to go over them in depth in this chapter, there are tutorials available at the website that will do so (see links in Additional Resources).

Future Value (FV)

This calculation can be used when setting goals. Essentially, if you input your current nest egg (PV), your expected rate of return (RATE), your ongoing annual contributions (PMT), and the length of time you will be saving (NPER), it will spit out how much money you will have in the end, i.e. the future value of your portfolio.

Present Value (PV)

This calculation is much less frequently used, but is essentially the future value calculation in reverse. If you want to know what the equivalent of a million dollars in 10 years would be today, you can use this calculation to arrive at that number.

Rate (RATE)

This calculation is a useful way to determine the rate of return on an investment or the interest rate on a debt. By inputting the present value, the future value, the period, and the payments, you can determine the rate.

Period (NPER)

This calculation allows you to determine how long it will take to reach a saving/investing goal or to pay off a debt. You input the present value, future value, rate, and payment and it will tell you the period, or length of time required to reach the goal.

Payment (PMT)

This calculation is particularly helpful for those trying to determine how much they want to save (or put toward a debt) in order to reach their goal in a certain time period.

As you can see, each of these five calculations are related to one another; you are simply solving for a different variable in the calculation each time. You can learn more about how to do these calculations at *www.whitecoatinvestor. com/compound-interest-the-excel-future-value-fv-function/*.

Principal Payment (PPMT)

Another useful calculation is the Principal Payment calculation. This is useful for people paying off a debt. As you are probably aware, when you first start paying on a mortgage, most of your payment goes toward interest. Toward the end of the mortgage, most of that payment is now going toward principal. This calculation tells you how much of any given payment is going toward principal. It is most useful if you run it after running the PMT calculation above. For example, if you had a 5%, 30-year, $100,000 loan, you would see that you would have to pay $6,505 per year. Then you could run the Principal Payment calculation and see that in the first year, $1,505 (or 23%) of your payment went toward principal. The rest went toward interest. However, in year 20, $3,803 (or 58%) of that $6,505 went toward principal. If doing that calculation does not convince you to pay a little extra on your loans each month, nothing will.

Annualized Rate of Return (XIRR)

This is the most complex of the calculations discussed in this section, but is still very useful when you want to know the true annualized return on your investments. By inputting all of the cash flows (money put into or taken out of the investment) along with the dates of each of those cash flows, you can see exactly how your investment is performing. I have been surprised how many times this number differs from the reported return given to me by those managing my investments. There is a tutorial on using this function at *www.whitecoatinvestor.com/how-to-calculate-your-return-the-excel-xirr-function/*.

RULES OF THUMB

I would like to finish this chapter by discussing some rules of thumb, each connected to a number. Like any rule of thumb, there are exceptions and nuances to each of these rules, but they are widely used in personal finance so it can be handy to be aware of them.

The first number I would like to discuss is 1%. There are two "rules" associated with this number. This first is the idea the financial services industry would like you to believe that 1% is the "standard rate" to manage money. 1% seems like a small number to most financial neophytes, but over long periods of time it can really add up. For example, over a 30-year time period paying just 1% in additional fees on a portfolio can mean having a 32% smaller nest egg. For a typical doctor, that can easily add up to a seven-figure amount. This rule should remind you to be mindful of fees, particularly ongoing fees based on a percentage of assets under management.

The other 1% rule is a rule that real estate investors use. It can be used as an initial screen for an income property. If you can charge 1% or more of the purchase price of a property as monthly rent, it is likely to "pencil out" as a good, cash-flowing rental property. Some investors even like to see monthly rents of 2%, although you are going to have a challenging time finding properties that even meet the 1% rule in many high cost-of-living areas with relatively high historical rates of appreciation.

The next "rule" I want you to be aware of is the 4% rule. This is a handy rule that can be used when setting goals for saving up a retirement nest egg. Using historical stock and bond return data, researchers have determined that a "safe withdrawal rate" (the amount of money, adjusted for inflation, that you can withdraw from a portfolio each year and expect it to last throughout a 30-year retirement without running out of money) is about 4%. The table on the next page is from the Trinity Study that best established this figure.[70] Using rolling 30-year periods of historical data and various mixes of stocks and bonds, they determined the "success rate" of the portfolio, that is how frequently the portfolio did not run out of money during a 30-year retirement.

So if you have a $1 million portfolio, you can withdraw $40,000 each year (4% x $1 million), adjusted each year for inflation. If you have a $2.5 million portfolio, you can withdraw $100,000 each year. This rule is most useful when used in reverse, i.e. multiplying your spending by 25 to determine your required nest egg size. If you calculate that you need $120,000 in retirement

Trinity Study

Retirement Portfolio Success Rates by Withdrawal Rate, Portfolio Composition, and Payout Period in Which Withdrawals Are Adjusted for Inflation

Annualized Withdrawal Rate as a Percentage of Initial Portfolio Value

Payout Period	3%	4%	5%	6%	7%	8%	9%	10%	11%	12%
100% Stocks										
15 Years	100%	100%	100%	94%	86%	76%	71%	64%	51%	46%
20 Years	100%	100%	100%	80%	72%	65%	52%	45%	38%	25%
25 Years	100%	100%	100%	88%	75%	63%	50%	42%	33%	17%
30 Years	100%	98%	80%	62%	55%	44%	33%	27%	15%	5%
75% Stocks/25% Bonds										
15 Years	100%	100%	100%	97%	87%	77%	70%	56%	47%	30%
20 Years	100%	100%	95%	80%	72%	60%	49%	31%	25%	11%
25 Years	100%	100%	87%	70%	58%	42%	32%	20%	10%	3%
30 Years	100%	100%	82%	60%	45%	35%	13%	5%	0%	0%
50% Stocks/50% Bonds										
15 Years	100%	100%	100%	99%	84%	71%	61%	44%	34%	21%
20 Years	100%	100%	94%	80%	63%	43%	31%	23%	8%	6%
25 Years	100%	100%	83%	60%	42%	23%	13%	8%	2%	2%
30 Years	100%	96%	67%	51%	22%	9%	0%	0%	0%	0%
25% Stocks/75% Bonds										
15 Years	100%	100%	100%	99%	77%	59%	43%	34%	26%	13%
20 Years	100%	100%	82%	52%	26%	14%	9%	3%	0%	0%
25 Years	100%	100%	58%	32%	25%	15%	8%	7%	2%	2%
30 Years	100%	80%	31%	22%	7%	0%	0%	0%	0%	0%
100% Bonds										
15 Years	100%	100%	100%	81%	54%	37%	37%	27%	19%	10%
20 Years	100%	97%	65%	37%	29%	28%	28%	8%	2%	2%
25 Years	100%	62%	33%	23%	18%	8%	8%	2%	2%	0%
30 Years	84%	35%	22%	11%	2%	0%	0%	0%	0%	0%

Note: Data for stock returns are monthly total returns to the Standard & Poor's 500 Index, and bond returns are total monthly returns to high-grade corporate bonds. Both sets of returns data are from January 1926 through December 2009 as published in the 2010 *Ibbotson SBBI Classic Yearbook* by Morningstar. Inflation adjustments were calculated using annual values of the CPI-U as published by the U.S. Bureau of Labor Statistics at www.bls.gov.

income from your nest egg each year, then you can quickly see that "your number" for financial independence is about $3 million. Many people feel this number should be a little lower given relatively low bond yields and expected stock returns (thus requiring a larger nest egg), but it should get you in the right neighborhood for basic calculations.

The 35% rule is one of my own that I find to be particularly useful for doctors. Many calculators and financial advisors use the 70% rule, meaning a retiree needs to replace 70% of their pre-retirement income in order to have the same standard of living in retirement as before. I find this estimate to be much too high for most doctors, which is a good thing since 70% of a doctor's salary during peak earnings years is a lot of money, especially once you multiply it by 25. The reason why 70% is too high is that many of the pre-retirement expenses of a doctor, especially a good saver, go away in retirement.

A typical doctor will pay dramatically less in taxes after retiring. Payroll taxes such as Social Security, Medicare, and even the PPACA specific taxes for most go away completely. Federal income taxes are dramatically reduced due to the progressive nature of the tax code. State income taxes go down even in a flat rate state and may go away completely if the retiree moves to a state without an income tax. It would not be unusual for a doctor to go from paying $100,000 in taxes to paying $10,000 in taxes after retiring. Another major expense that goes away in retirement is retirement savings. If you are saving 20% of your gross income for retirement as I recommend, you do not have to replace that in retirement. There is no more need to save at that point!

If you pay off your mortgage before retiring, that major expense also drops out of your budget. Disability and term life insurance policies can also be dropped now that you are financially independent, saving those premiums. Child-related expenses should go down dramatically once the children are out of the house. You also no longer need to save for their college. Work-related expenses (commuting costs, CME, malpractice insurance, work clothes, board certification fees, medical staff fees, licensing and DEA fees) also disappear. Every budget will be slightly different, but if you run these numbers for yourself, you will likely find that you only need your nest egg to replace 25–50% (or about 35%) of your pre-retirement income to maintain the same standard of living in retirement.

The 55% rule, another handy rule for real estate investors, contains a lesson for anyone buying a house. An experienced real estate investor knows that approximately 45% of the income for the property (i.e. the collected rent) will go toward non-mortgage expenses. These include property taxes, insurance, repairs, renovations, management fees, snow removal, lawn care, and vacancies, leaving 55% of the rent to divide between the mortgage and profit. Every property is different, but you know if the person selling the property to you is claiming that only 20% of rent goes toward expenses, something is wrong with the information. As a home buyer, you can also see that just because the mortgage is less than renting an equivalent place does not mean you should buy a home. There are a lot more expenses associated with homeownership than just the mortgage principal and interest. Too many doctors do not learn this lesson until their second or third home purchase.

Our final rule of thumb worth learning is the Rule of 72. This handy rule demonstrates the power of compound interest. You can use it to determine how quickly your money (or debt) will double at a given rate of return (or interest rate). For example, if your money is growing at 2% per year, it will require 72/2 = 36 years to double. If your money is growing at 7.2%, it will require 10 years to double. If you can increase your rate of return to 10% per year, your money will double every 7.2 years. Interest on debt is just compound interest in reverse. For example, if you borrow at 20% (and do not make any payments), in 72/20 = 3.6 years you will owe twice as much money. The calculation is not perfect, but it is close enough to be a useful rule of thumb.

Becoming financially literate requires the ability to do basic math, the use of a financial calculator or spreadsheet, and the knowledge of some basic personal finance rules of thumb. Unfortunately, so few people in our modern society are both financially literate and financially disciplined that if you can manage to be both it may feel like a superpower.

MAIN IDEAS

- The math required to be a personal finance ace is not particularly complicated.

- Know your net worth, income, marginal tax rate, effective tax rate, and savings rate.

- Knowing how to use a financial calculator or the financial functions of a spreadsheet is an important part of being financially literate.

ADDITIONAL RESOURCES

- **Resource:** Google Sheets, a Free Spreadsheet
  www.google.com/sheets/about/

- **Blog Post:** Future Value Function Tutorial
  www.whitecoatinvestor.com/compound-interest-the-excel-future-value-fv-function/

- **Blog Post:** How to Calculate Your Return—The XIRR Tutorial
  www.whitecoatinvestor.com/how-to-calculate-your-return-the-excel-xirr-function/

- **Blog Post:** The 4% Rule
  www.whitecoatinvestor.com/the-4-rule-safe-withdrawal-rates/

- **Blog Post:** The Rule of 72
  www.whitecoatinvestor.com/the-rule-of-72-understanding-compound-interest/

- **Resource:** Moneychimp Calculators
  www.moneychimp.com/calculator/

AN INVITATION

Congratulations! You have accomplished a feat that is surprisingly rare among doctors. You have successfully read a financial book! Along the way, I hope you have learned a few things that you can implement now, made plans to take important financial steps in the future, and been inspired to reach the financial success you deserve. As you continue to learn and apply the concepts learned here in your life, you will continually become more successful at all of the monetary tasks of life, including earning, saving, investing, spending, and giving.

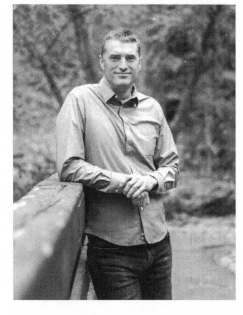

This is the point in my book where I trust you with my email address. Over the years, readers have emailed me praise, criticism, comments, and questions. I have assisted them in finding the resources they needed in their lives. Sometimes this is simply information, and I can point them to a blog post or podcast I have already produced. Other times, they need the assistance of a professional. I maintain a list of professionals under the "Recommended" tab on *The White Coat Investor* website. This includes student loan refinancing companies, student loan coaches, mortgage lenders, independent insurance agents, financial advisors, real estate investing companies, attorneys, accountants, realtors, and more. If you need these services, please check out those lists. These partners have been vetted by me and thousands of readers over the years.

At the website you will also find additional resources, including recommended books, online courses, our podcast, our videocast, and our forums, Subreddit, and Facebook Group. You can learn about the live Continuing Medical Education eligible Physician Wellness and Financial Literacy conferences we put on. Information can also be found there about the WCI Scholarship (why not apply?) and the WCI Financial Educator award.

If you are having trouble finding what you need, or just want to say hi, shoot me an email at editor@whitecoatinvestor.com. So far, I have been able to respond personally to every single reader who has emailed me and I hope to continue to do so for years to come.

Now that I have trusted you with my email address, I want you to trust me with yours. If you will do so, I will not spam you and you can unsubscribe at any time. You can sign up for our free monthly newsletter (includes a market report and a super-secret blog post not found anywhere else) and our WCI Boot Camp email series. You can even get every blog post I publish in your email box. As if all that is not enough, if you will sign up at *www.whitecoatinvestor.com/bonus*, I will send you four bonus chapters for this book in PDF form. If you enjoyed the four "Financial Literacy 100" chapters, you are really going to like these. I call them the "Financial Literacy 200" chapters, and they include:

Financial Literacy 201: Interacting with Financial Advisors

Financial Literacy 202: Insurance

Financial Literacy 203: Contract Review and Negotiation

Financial Literacy 204: Real Estate Investing

SIGN UP NOW

AN INVITATION

You will find this information invaluable as you move into your career. Each is packed with life-changing information you need to know, but nobody at your school is going to teach you.

I have one last favor to ask you. The more book reviews that a book gets, the more people Amazon shows the book to. In order to help get this valuable information into the hands of even more students like you, I would appreciate it if you would leave a five-star review on Amazon for it. Thank you in advance.

WRITE A REVIEW NOW

I hope you have found this book to be valuable. It was created with the medical or dental student in mind. I am so thankful for the motivation, compassion, and hard work that has driven you into this career. I want to see you succeed in your practice and your finances. We have walked together through the important financial decisions you will make during school and the early years of your residency. We have discussed the most critical aspects of financial literacy for doctors. Now it is time to implement what you have learned in your life. You can do it. Along with the entire White Coat Investor community, I will be right by your side every step of the way.

Jim Dahle, MD

Founder, The White Coat Investor
www.whitecoatinvestor.com

ACKNOWLEDGMENTS

I would have expected that it would have been easier to write a third book than either of the first two, but it seems that each book requires more effort! This one would not have been possible without the support of so many.

A special thank you goes to my beloved Katie and four children; without their support, there would be no White Coat Investor at all.

To the rest of the staff here at WCI—I told you I would get this book done eventually! Seriously though, thanks for your gentle teasing to help push me through when motivation waned. As you know, I would have quit this entire enterprise long ago without your support. Thank you for putting up with the worst boss in the world.

Thank you to Rick Ferri, CFA, not only for writing the foreword and providing support for WCI over the years, but also for writing books that influenced me so much years ago.

Readers may not be aware that the first drafts of my books are never anywhere near as good as the published version. The main reason why is the volunteer army of reviewers willing to tear it to pieces so it can be built back up properly. Thank you to the following individuals who reviewed the manuscript and offered helpful suggestions, most of which were incorporated into the book: Brett Stevens, MBA; Warner Weber; Gwendolyn A. Quintana, MPH, MS4; Col. Gregory Morgan, Ret. USAF, CPA; Alexandra E. Forest, DDS, MD; Mitchell D. Belkin, medical student; Jake Babel, OMS4; Kolten Astle, dental student; Jonathan Polak, MD; Chris Roff, dental student; Katherine Y. Lee, DO, MPH; J. Lee Rawlings, MD; Austin Snyder, medical student; Mujtaba A. Hameed, medical student; Angela Chiara, MA, dental student; Brigid Cruser, MS2; Nicholas Cozzi, MD, MBA; Anas M. Saad, MD; Chelsea G. Swanson, JD; Dr. Craig & Ashley Weinstein; Mary Cruser; Maksim Vaysman, DO, MS; and Ryan Kelly, CFP.

NOTES

INTRODUCTION

1. "Historical Consumer Price Index (CPI-U) Data," Inflation Data, Tim McMahon, accessed December 26, 2020, https://inflationdata.com/Inflation/Consumer_Price_Index/HistoricalCPI.aspx?reloaded=true.

2. Erik Sherman, "College Tuition Is Rising at Twice the Inflation Rate—While Students Learn at Home," *Forbes*, August 31, 2020, https://www.forbes.com/sites/zengernews/2020/08/31/college-tuition-is-rising-at-twice-the-inflation-rate-while-students-learn-at-home/?sh=5ba1026a2f98.

3. "Tuition and Student Fees Reports," AAMC, accessed December 26, 2020, https://www.aamc.org/data-reports/reporting-tools/report/tuition-and-student-fees-reports.

4. Leslie Kane, "Medscape Physician Debt and Net Worth Report 2020," *Medscape*, June 24, 2020, https://www.medscape.com/slideshow/2020-compensation-debt-worth-6012988.

CHAPTER 1

5. Sarah Butcher, "Pay in Banking vs. Consulting vs. Tech vs. Medicine vs. Law," *eFinancialCareers*, January 15, 2020, https://www.efinancialcareers.com/news/2020/01/pay-in-banking-vs-consulting-vs-tech-vs-medicine-vs-law.

CHAPTER 2

6. Dave Ramsey, "Don't Be Stupid About How You Pay for Education," The Dave Ramsey Show, September 26, 2016, https://youtu.be/NxrcHcYBNe4.

7. "Graduation Questionnire (GQ)," AAMC, accessed December 26, 2020, https://www.aamc.org/data-reports/students-residents/report/graduation-questionnaire-gq.

8. "AACOM Reports: Entering and Graduating Class Surveys," American Association of Colleges of Osteopathic Medicine (AACOM), accessed December 26, 2020, https://www.aacom.org/reports-programs-initiatives/aacom-reports/entering-and-graduating-class-surveys.

9. "ADEA Survey of Dental School Seniors, 2018 Graduating Class Tables Report," ADEA: The Voice of Dental Education, November 2018, https://www.adea.org/data/seniors/.

10. Josh Mitchell, "Mike Meru Has $1 Million in Student Loans. How Did That Happen?," *The Wall Street Journal*, May 25, 2018, https://www.wsj.com/articles/mike-meru-has-1-million-in-student-loans-how-did-that-happen-1527252975.

CHAPTER 3

11. "Results and Data: 2019 Main Residency Match," The Match: National Resident Matching Program, May 2019, https://www.nrmp.org/main-residency-match-data/.

12. "2013–2021 Tuition and Student Fees Reports," AAMC, accessed December 26, 2020, https://www.aamc.org/data-reports/reporting-tools/report/tuition-and-student-fees-reports.

13. "Osteopathic College Tuition and Fees (1st Year) 2020–2021 and Historical," American Association of Colleges of Osteopathic Medicine (AACOM), accessed December 26, 2020, https://www.aacom.org/reports-programs-initiatives/aacom-reports/tuition-fees-and-financial-aid.

14. "Dental School Rankings," The Student Doctor Network (SDN), accessed December 26, 2020, https://www.studentdoctor.net/schools/schools/3/dental-school-rankings/0.

CHAPTER 4

15. Devasmita Chakraverty, Donna B. Jeffe, and Robert H. Tai, "Transition Experiences in MD-PhD Programs,"*CBE Life Sciences Education* 17, no. 3 (Fall 2018): ar41, https://www.ncbi.nlm.nih.gov/pmc/articles/PMC6234812/.

CHAPTER 6

16. Ecclesiastes 3:1, 2, 6 (KJV).

CHAPTER 7

17. "2019 MSQ All Schools Summary Report (PDF)," AAMC, accessed December 26, 2020, https://www.aamc.org/data-reports/students-residents/report/matriculating-student-questionnaire-msq.

CHAPTER 8

18. Internal data from a White Coat Investor social media poll.

19. Leslie Kane, "Medscape Physician Compensation Report 2020," *Medscape*, May 14, 2020, https://www.medscape.com/slideshow/2020-compensation-overview-6012684.

20. American College of Emergency Physicians, and Daniel Stern and Associates, *2015 National Emergency Medicine Salary Survey: Clinical Results* (Irving, TX: American College of Emergency Physicians, 2015).

CHAPTER 9

21. Internal data from a White Coat Investor social media poll. Similar "@WCInvestor" Twitter poll and data can be seen at https://www.whitecoatinvestor.com/wp-content/uploads/2020/10/Screen-Shot-2020-10-23-at-9.10.17-AM-1.png.

22. Jonathan Clements, *How to Think About Money* (CreateSpace Independent Publishing Platform, 2016). https:amzn.to/38FKEKe.

23. "Health Policy Institute: Income and Gross Billings," American Dental Association (ADA), accessed January 2020, https://www.ada.org/en/science-research/health-policy-institute/dental-statistics/income-billing-and-other-dentistry-statistics.

24. "Dental Match Statistics: Phase | Summary Charts," National Matching Services Inc., accessed December 28, 2020, https://natmatch.com/dentres/stats/statistics-summary-ph1.html.

25. "Dental Match Statistics: Summary Statistics," National Matching Services Inc., accessed December 28, 2020, https://natmatch.com/dentres/stats/statistics-summary.html.

CHAPTER 10

26. Sylvie Stacy, *50 Nonclinical Careers for Physicians: Fulfilling, Meaningful, and Lucrative Alternatives to Direct Patient Care* (American Association for Physician Leadership, 2020). https:amzn.to/2URrrie.

27. "Main Residency Match Data and Reports," The Match: National Residency Matching Program, accessed December 28, 2020, https://www.nrmp.org/main-residency-match-data/.

CHAPTER 11

28. Sara Berg, "WHO Adds Burnout to ICD-11. What It Means for Physicians," *AMA,* July 23, 2019, https://www.ama-assn.org/practice-management/physician-health/who-adds-burnout-icd-11-what-it-means-physicians.

29. Richard A. Friedman, "Is Burnout Real?," *The New York Times*, June 3, 2019,
    https://www.nytimes.com/2019/06/03/opinion/burnout-stress.html.

30. Nadia Goodman, "How Google's Marissa Mayer Prevents Burnout," *Entrepreneur*, June 6, 2012,
    https://www.entrepreneur.com/article/223723.

31. Leslie Kane, "Medscape National Physician Burnout and Suicide Report 2020: The Generational Divide," *Medscape*, January 15, 2020,
    https://www.medscape.com/slideshow/2020-lifestyle-burnout-6012460.

32. Internal data from a White Coat Investor social media poll. Similar "@WCInvestor" Twitter poll and data can be seen at https://www.whitecoatinvestor.com/wp-content/uploads/2020/10/Screen-Shot-2020-10-23-at-9.10.17-AM-1.png.

CHAPTER 12

33. "Main Residency Match Data and Reports," The Match: National Residency Matching Program, accessed December 28, 2020,
    https://www.nrmp.org/main-residency-match-data/.

CHAPTER 13

34. Carol Kane, "2018 Benchmark Survey: Updated Data on Physician Practice Arrangements: For the First Time, Fewer Physicians Are Owners than Employees," *AMA: Policy Research Perspectives*, 2018,
    https://www.ama-assn.org/system/files/2019-07/prp-fewer-owners-benchmark-survey-2018.pdf.

35. Michelle Manchir, "Practice Ownership Declining Among Dentists," *ADA News*, August 30, 2017,
    https://www.ada.org/en/publications/ada-news/2017-archive/august/practice-ownership-declining-among-dentists.

36. "Health Policy Institute: Income and Gross Billings," American Dental Association (ADA), accessed January 2020,
    https://www.ada.org/en/science-research/health-policy-institute/dental-statistics/income-billing-and-other-dentistry-statistics.

CHAPTER 14

37. Summarized from Ecclesiastes 3:1 (KJV).

CHAPTER 16

38. Jonathan Clements, "How to Think About Money as a Physician" (speech), March 3, 2018, Physician Wellness and Financial Literacy Conference—Park City, video available in the conference course found at https://whitecoatinvestor.teachable.com/p/physician-wellness-and-financial-literacy-conference-park-city.

39. Matt Krantz, "24 Bankruptcies Prove You Can Lose 90% of Your Money on Stocks," *Investor's Business Daily*, May 7, 2020, https://www.investors.com/etfs-and-funds/sectors/bankrupt-companies-prove-you-can-lose-90-percent-money-stocks/.

40. Berlinda Liu, "SPIVA U.S. Year-End 2019 Scorecard: Active Funds Continued to Lag," *S&P Global*, April 8, 2020, https://www.spglobal.com/en/research-insights/articles/spiva-u-s-year-end-2019-scorecard-active-funds-continued-to-lag.

CHAPTER 19

41. "Earnings Release FY19 Q4," Microsoft, July 18, 2019, https://www.microsoft.com/en-us/Investor/earnings/FY-2019-Q4/press-release-webcast.

42. "List of Countries by GDP (Nominal)," Wikipedia, accessed December 28, 2020, https://en.wikipedia.org/wiki/List_of_countries_by_GDP_(nominal).

43. "GDP by State," Bureau of Economic Analysis (BEA): U.S. Department of Commerce, accessed December 28, 2020, https://www.bea.gov/data/gdp/gdp-state.

44. Benjamin Graham, in discussion with Warren Buffet, quoted in Warren E. Buffet, "Letter to the Shareholders of Berkshire Hathaway Inc.," Berkshire Hathaway Inc., March 1, 1994, https://www.berkshirehathaway.com/letters/1993.html.

45. "Sectors and Industries Overview," Fidelity Investments, January 2020, https://eresearch.fidelity.com/eresearch/markets_sectors/sectors/sectors_in_market.jhtml.

46. Vanguard, *Vanguard Total Stock Market Index Fund Summary Prospectus*, April 28, 2020, 2–3, https://advisors.vanguard.com/pub/Pdf/sp85.pdf.

CHAPTER 20

47. "IRS Provides Tax Inflation Adjustments for Tax Year 2021," IRS, October 26, 2020, https://www.irs.gov/newsroom/irs-provides-tax-inflation-adjustments-for-tax-year-2021.

48. "Historical Highest Marginal Income Tax Rates," Tax Policy Center (TPC): Urban Institute and Brookings Institution, February 4, 2020, https://www.taxpolicycenter.org/statistics/historical-highest-marginal-income-tax-rates.

49. Robert McClelland and Nikhita Airi, "Effective Income Tax Rates Have Fallen for the Top One Percent Since World War II," Tax Policy Center (TPC): Urban Institute and Brookings Institution, January 6, 2020, https://www.taxpolicycenter.org/taxvox/effective-income-tax-rates-have-fallen-top-one-percent-world-war-ii.

CHAPTER 21

50. Recommended resources to learn more about financial history: William J. Bernstein, *The Four Pillars of Investing: Lessons for Building a Winning Portfolio* (McGraw-Hill Education, 2010). https://amzn.to/37SyPRZ.
Charles Mackay, *Extraordinary Popular Delusions and the Madness of Crowds* (CreateSpace Independent Publishing Platform, 2016). https://amzn.to/37VawD5.
Andrew H. Browning, *The Panic of 1819: The First Great Depression* (University of Missouri, 2019). https://amzn.to/37TjIaL.

51. Attributed to Mark Twain, https://quoteinvestigator.com/2014/01/12/history-rhymes/.

52. G.R. Driver and John C. Miles, *The Babylonian Laws* (The Clarendon Press, 1955).

53. Cyrus H. Gordon, *Hammurapi's Code* (Holt, Reinhart and Winston, 1965), 8.

54. Bava Metzia, fol. 42, col. 1.

55. Isaac Newton, quoted in John O'Farrell, *An Utterly Impartial History of Britain or 2000 Years of Upper-Class Idiots in Charge* (Doubleday, 2007). https://amzn.to/3rAyiMl.

56. John Rothchild, "When the Shoeshine Boys Talk Stocks It Was a Great Sell Signal in 1929. So What Are the Shoeshine Boys Talking About Now?," *Fortune Magazine*, April 15, 1996, https://archive.fortune.com/magazines/fortune/fortune_archive/1996/04/15/211503/index.htm.

57. Evelyn Cheng, "Bitcoin Is Not a Classic Bubble, But Still Be 'Suspicious,' Says Investing Expert William Bernstein," *CNBC*, October 24, 2017, https://www.cnbc.com/2017/10/24/william-bernstein-bitcoin-is-not-a-classic-bubble.html.

58. James K. Glassman and Kevin A. Hassett, *Dow 36,000: The New Strategy for Profiting from the Coming Rise in the Stock Market* (Three Rivers Press, 2000). https://amzn.to/2WTjz0M.

59. Dan Murphy, "Analyst Who Predicted Bitcoin's Rise Now Sees It Hitting $300,000–$400,000," *CNBC*, December 17, 2017, https://www.cnbc.com/2017/12/17/bitcoin-price-ronnie-moas-sees-cryptocurrency-at-300000-400000.html.

60. William J. Bernstein, *Deep Risk: How History Informs Portfolio Design* (Efficient Frontier Advisors, 2013). https://amzn.to/2WOyU2A.

61. "List of Nationalizations by Country," Wikipedia, accessed December 28, 2020, https://en.wikipedia.org/wiki/List_of_nationalizations_by_country.

62. "The Callan Periodic Table of Investment Returns 2000–2019," Callan Institute, 2020, https://www.callan.com/wp-content/uploads/2020/01/Classic-Periodic-Table.pdf.

63. John C. Bogle, *Common Sense on Mutual Funds: Fully Updated 10th Anniversary Edition* (J. Wiley & Sons, 2010). https://amzn.to/2WM0ail.

64. "Compound Annual Growth Rate (Annualized Return)," Moneychimp, accessed December 28, 2020, http://www.moneychimp.com/features/market_cagr.htm.

65. "Vanguard Portfolio Allocation Models," Vanguard, accessed December 28, 2020, https://personal.vanguard.com/us/insights/saving-investing/model-portfolio-allocations.

66. Jeremy Siegel, *Stocks for the Long Run 5/E: The Definitive Guide to Financial Market Returns & Long-Term Investment Strategies* (McGraw-Hill Education, 2014). https://amzn.to/2WM0ail.

67. "Federal Funds Rate—62 Year Historical Chart," Macrotrends, accessed December 28, 2020, https://www.macrotrends.net/2015/fed-funds-rate-historical-chart.

68. "Historical Highest Marginal Income Tax Rates," Tax Policy Center (TPC): Urban Institute and Brookings Institution, February 4, 2020, https://www.taxpolicycenter.org/statistics/historical-highest-marginal-income-tax-rates.

CHAPTER 22

69. Morgan Housel, *The Psychology of Money: Timeless Lessons on Wealth, Greed, and Happiness* (Harriman House, 2020). https://amzn.to/38HZPTf.

70. Philip L. Cooley, Carl M. Hubbard, and Daniel T. Walz, "Retirement Savings: Choosing a Withdrawal Rate That Is Sustainable," *Journal of the American Association of Individual Investors* (February 1998): 16–21, https://www.aaii.com/journal/199802/feature.pdf.

Made in the USA
Middletown, DE
07 May 2021